Kathleen Burns, MFT

Learning and Teaching Therapy

The Guilford Family Therapy Series
Michael P. Nichols, *Series Editor*

LEARNING AND TEACHING THERAPY

Jay Haley

THE GUILFORD PRESS
New York London

©1996 The Guilford Press
A Division of Guilford Publications, Inc.
72 Spring Street, New York, NY 10012

Printed in the United States of America

This book is printed on acid-free paper.

Last digit is print number: 9 8 7 6 5 4 3 2

Library of Congress Cataloging-in-Publication Data
Haley, Jay.
    Learning and teaching therapy / by Jay Haley.
        p. cm.—(The Guilford family therapy series)
    Includes bibliographical references and index.
    ISBN 1-57230-035-3
    1. Psychotherapy—Study and teaching. 2. Psychotherapists
—Supervision of. 3. Psychotherapy—Study and teaching
—Supervision. I. Title. II. Series.
RC459.H35 1996
616.89'14'0711—dc20   95-50953
                                                        CIP

To my wife, Maddy

PREFACE

When one learns to drive a car, there are consequences if one does it badly. Therefore, it is best to have an experienced driver sit with the beginner for driving practice, ready to take over if there is difficulty on the street. Beginners are taught the rules of the road as well as the skills involved in driving the vehicle. Before they can ride solo, they are given a written test and then a driving test, which means that their ability to follow all the rules of the road and park the car is actually observed. When the test is passed, the trainee is officially a licensed driver. Still, passing the driving test doesn't mean one can drive and park a truck, and some drivers won't be able to drive a stick shift. It is experience on the road that increases one's skills.

Suppose one learned how to drive by having a teacher discuss different makes of cars and how it feels to become a driver. The student would never be observed driving, and there would be no practice with an experienced driver ready to take over if need be. There would be no driving test to pass. The teacher, who would have no responsibility for the actions of the trainee on the road, would simply give the student the keys and wish him or her luck.

Surely, no sensible learner would wish to be taught that way. Should we take learning therapy as seriously as we take learning to drive a car?

HOW IS THERAPY TAUGHT?

During the first hundred years of psychotherapy, trainees primarily learned therapy by undergoing it themselves. It was assumed that having personal therapy would create a competent therapist. In addition, there were conversations or seminars on the reasons why people behave strangely; these were often philosophical discussions about the nature of man. The trainee was never observed or recorded doing therapy. Training was an apprenticeship in which the apprentice never observed the master at work and the master never observed the apprentice.

In a training program the teacher didn't take responsibility for a trainee's failure with a case (since the teacher couldn't see what was happening, responsibility could hardly be taken). Nor was there a test or evaluation of the trainee's ability. What actually happened in a therapy case was not known. When therapists encountered a tragic development with a case and returned to the teacher for counsel, they would be asked how they felt about this tragedy, and their personal reactions would be examined. They would then be wished good luck and sent forth to the next client—or the next tragedy.

TRAINING TODAY

The task of therapists today is to learn therapy by taking it as seriously as they would take learning to drive a car. Therapy training is not philosophical discussions on the nature of man. It is learning interview skills and therapeutic techniques for the variety of clients who seek help, techniques that must be practiced. If a trainee is taught badly, many people will suffer the consequences. In this age of managed care, false memories, and malpractice suits, trainees risk being taken to court if they don't know what they are doing. Even the supervisor can be taken to court. This situation increases the concern about training people to be competent. We also inherit each other's failures. If we fail with a case, it makes things more difficult for the next therapist dealing with that person.

When one is teaching a skill, like driving a car, it seems obvious that the practice should be observed. A therapist should be guided through the complexities of a case. To do that, the teacher must know what is actually happening. The therapist must learn what to do to change people, and how to put that learning into practice. Basic training is required, whatever one's philosophy.

As we enter the second hundred years of psychotherapy the technology available to us for observing and recording therapy sessions involves audio- and videotapes as well as one-way mirrors. Teachers and therapists are no longer trapped by a single method of therapy or stultifying diagnostic categories. They are now free to innovate, though one hopes the desire to establish new schools of therapy will be restrained. What should be taught are the techniques for conducting successful therapy: how to ask a question, make a comment, give a directive, determine who should be in an interview, and plan the strategy of a case.

ACKNOWLEDGMENTS

Thirty years ago I published *Strategies of Psychotherapy*. It was a product of Gregory Bateson's project on communication. The primary emphasis was on describing psychopathology as a form of communication and therapy as a way of deliberately changing that communication. This view required thinking of people in terms of units of two or more and so introduced therapy concepts and practices that differ from those based on an emphasis on the individual's thought processes. The social milieu of the client became the focus of therapy. What had to change was the way therapists were trained, and this required the overcoming of immense inertia. The present book expresses my views of training based on 30 years of experience in teaching the art of changing people.

I was never formally trained as a clinician in a particular profession. Since I had no investment in a particular therapy ideology, I think it was easier for me to change my thinking about therapy. I was also influenced, if not supervised, by several extraordinary people. Gregory Bateson was not enthusiastic about changing people; he was an anthropologist and preferred to study them. Yet he was a fountain of ideas that were relevant to the field of psychotherapy and its changes. Working with him full time for 10 years, investigating whatever I wished, was a unique research experience. I shared this experience with John Weakland, whose influence on me was invaluable. Like Bateson, his thinking wasn't trapped by orthodoxy in the field of anthropology.

Another extraordinary person who had a major influence on my thinking about therapy was Milton H. Erickson. From him I learned therapeutic technique as well as a practical view of life and human problems. With Weakland I studied Erickson's communicative view of hypnosis. When I went into practice, I consulted Erickson about cases over the years, thus learning a great deal about his unique approach to therapy. He also became a model for me while I was searching for a posture for being a therapist.

A great support for me, particularly in relation to psychiatry and schizophrenia, was Don Jackson. He was the psychiatric consultant on the Bateson project. Quite different from Erickson in his approach, he held the same practical view of human dilemmas. Jackson was the West Coast authority on schizophrenia and remarkably successful in therapy with schizophrenics. He believed there was nothing wrong with a schizophrenic that wasn't a response to his or her social situation. It was remarkable to observe Jackson doing therapy with psychotic people; his attitude was that they were curable and that nothing was physiologically wrong with them. He was one of the best clinicians I've seen, particularly in his skill with schizophrenics and their families. Unfortunately, he died young, apparently accidentally, from an overdose of medication.

Many of Jackson's ideas came from Harry Stack Sullivan, who personally supervised him at Chestnut Lodge. In the 1960s the Group for the Advancement of Psychiatry surveyed a sample of family therapists and found that a surprising number of them had some connection with Sullivan, even though he himself did not interview whole families. Sullivan's idea that in individual therapy there are two people in the room reflected his belief that the therapist isn't just a blank screen onto which the patient projects fantasies. When I reported a patient's verbalization to Jackson, his supervisory question to me (as Sullivan's had been to him) was, "What were you doing just before the patient said that?" Psychotic behavior was assumed to be responsive behavior, like all other behavior in therapy.

There was another extraordinary individual I had the good fortune to associate with in the 1950s: Alan Watts. An authority on Zen Buddhism, he was an informal consultant to our project because of our shared interest in paradox. He introduced the ideas of Zen, which we could see as an alternate therapy and as a welcome alternative to psychodynamic ideology in that period. For a thousand years Zen included the experience of one person trying to change another, a change brought about not by insight into oneself or by conversation or free association but by actions and directives, with the goal being to live by experiencing and not by monitoring oneself.

I also learned from Salvador Minuchin, with whom I worked for almost 10 years. He, the creative Braulio Montalvo, and I shared an enthusiasm for the new developments in therapy during the 1960s. We spent many hours discussing therapy and how to train therapists in different fields, as well as nonprofessionals.

None of these teachers, to whom I owe a great debt, were orthodox members of their professions. Bateson was not quite accepted in the anthropological world, and Erickson, Jackson, and Minuchin were outside the mainstream in the fields of psychotherapy, psychiatry, and child psychiatry, respectively; Watts was what he called "backdoor Zen." Moreover, none of them taught in academia, except for marginal classes. Yet out of their divergent views came a family-oriented brief therapy that many academics are now trying to teach in the universities. Apparently, the methods of training therapists change more slowly than the practices of therapy. This may be primarily because therapists wish to teach what their teachers taught. In times of rapid change in ideology and practice, this tendency becomes a problem.

An acknowledgment section presents difficulties since I owe so much to so many colleagues and students. I have been to hundreds of meetings where ideas were exchanged with colleagues. I also learned a great deal from the hundreds of people I have trained. Many of my trainees, such as Neil Schiff, whom I have enjoyed working with over the years, have become colleagues and fellow supervisors. To list some people as contributors to the ideas in this book would mean neglecting others, and there are so many who are participating in the development of current ideas in the therapy field.

I also wish to express my appreciation to Michael Nichols, whose editorial consultation did much to improve this work.

CONTENTS

1

TEACHING THERAPY

Today is an exciting time in the field of therapy because everything is changing. There is no orthodoxy. Without orthodoxy no one can conform and no one can be a deviant. There is no right way of doing therapy, only different ways. You can create a new therapy technique, or revive an old one, and not be thought of as heretical. In fact, if you give the technique a name, you may even initiate a new school of therapy and conduct workshops.

One might think that after 100 years there would be consensus in therapy, that there would be agreement on how to formulate a client's problem and how to intervene to make a change. However, there is not even agreement that clinicians should attempt to formulate the problem presented by a client, make an intervention, or deliberately try to change the client.

Beginning in the 1950s, with the development of communication and behavioral ideas, orthodoxy weakened, and a banquet of different therapy approaches began to emerge. This process is continuing, with many consequences to the field, particularly in training. In this time of change everyone becomes either a teacher or a trainee since the techniques that are being developed on the basis of new premises must be learned by every practitioner who wants to stay current. New skills are required in therapy interviewing, new ways of financing therapy must be adapted to, and new types of clients are arriving. There is also a new focus on brief therapy; long-term therapy is out of fashion.

As therapy changes, many supervisors are no longer leading the field but are themselves trying to catch up with what's happening. Often they must unlearn their past training while trying to teach new approaches based on opposite premises. Those teachers who were trained in orthodoxy risk the condemnation of their own teachers if they change, a situation many find painful. Trainees find the diversity confusing as they discover that many of their teachers disagree with each other. As they go from workshop to workshop, hoping to learn what to do with their desperate clients, many trainees, disappointed with what they find, decide they must devise their own approach to therapy.

One of the major changes in therapy now taking place is the pressure on the trainee therapist to learn to deal with all sorts of problems. To survive today a therapist must be a generalist, not a specialist. In the past a therapist would specialize in children's problems, or marital problems, or eating disorders. With the new ways of financing therapy through managed care, therapists must be able to deal with whatever problem comes in the door. They can no longer choose among cases, referring out the ones they don't specialize in. A therapist in private practice today must deal with many different kinds of problems to have enough cases for the turnover inherent in today's brief therapy. After working in an agency devoted to the treatment of one type of symptomatic client, therapists can find themselves unable to move to another agency whose clients have a different set of problems unless they have been properly trained to treat a variety of cases. Training programs must try to provide trainee therapists with the experience of treating clients of every type, and supervisors cannot afford to confine their teaching to the treatment of a single type of client but must be able to provide instruction on the treatment of many different types.

Learning to be a therapist doesn't mean merely learning a set of skills, as one would with carpentry. The instrument of change in therapy is the therapist, and that instrument can be uncertain or faulty. It's the supervisor's job not only to teach therapists *what* to do but to help them when they find themselves with personal reactions that keep them from functioning as they should. Trainee therapists are asked to respond to, and change, human beings in distress when in their naivete they may find the problem presented to be unbelievable. (Other problems may be familiar to them from their own experiences.)

Trainees might find in this book an approach that is different from, if not critical of, the approach of their supervisors. Such differences aren't made to make trouble but to correct ideas and procedures. I'm reminded of a long-ago conversation that took place after I wrote "The Art of Psychoanalysis."[1] I showed the manuscript to Donald Jackson, asking him if he thought it might upset people in analysis and interfere with their progress. Jackson replied that a competent analyst could handle this issue

---

[1]Haley, J. (1958). The art of psychoanalysis. *ETC, 15,* 190–200.

and one should not protect incompetent analysts. I think the same consideration applies here to supervisors.

I hope this book will help clinicians who are learning therapy, teaching therapy, or practicing in these changing times. Therapists learn to change people, and in the process they often change themselves. The supervisor serves as a guide to achieve those ends. When dealing with a case, the trainee focuses on the client, while the supervisor focuses on both the client and the trainee. While concerned about the needs of the client, the supervisor must also consider what the trainee knows and how to enlarge his or her range of skills. The supervisor might know several ways to approach various symptoms; the one chosen should help the client change and also help increase the trainee's experience with therapy interventions.

Supervisors must teach trainee therapists to be skillful tacticians while responding sensitively to a client's misery and distress. Supervising is the teaching not only of techniques of therapy but also of an appreciation and understanding of tragic human dilemmas. Therapists must become experts in helping clients, which can be taught, but they must also be sensitive and human, which perhaps cannot be taught.

Some trainees become so immersed in theories that they seem inhuman. For example, I once visited an academic setting for the presentation of an interview by two young therapists who were pleased with their knowledge and wished to show me how well they were learning to do therapy. It was a first interview with a couple and their two adolescent children (who had come reluctantly). After seating the family, the two therapists told them that they would like to begin by explaining their approach. The family seemed agreeable to that. The therapists, taking turns speaking, said they preferred cotherapy because "two heads are better than one." They explained that cotherapy prevents therapists from siding with one member of the family and being unfair to the others, since the two therapists can correct each other. They also said that at times they might disagree with each other but that this would show families how to deal with disagreements. The family members nodded in understanding.

The therapists went on to say that they prefer to see the whole family in the first interview so that they can see the family system in action. After explaining that all family members would have a chance to speak and express their individual views, they pointed out that some therapists prefer to focus on the individual instead of the whole family. Their own approach did not mean, they said, that they were blaming the family for an individual member's problems but only that they believed that since all family members participate in family life, they can be helpful in understanding and solving the problem of an individual member. They then proceeded to explain systems theory (at times correcting each other), emphasizing that they were necessarily leaving out the full complexity of it. This presentation by the young therapists of their theory and approach lasted 25 minutes—until the supervisor interrupted and suggested that they ask the family why they were there.

TWO EXTREME VIEWS OF THERAPY

Ways of teaching therapy differ with the ideology and approach of a particular school of thought. The approach recommended here is designed for a therapy that is brief and active that takes into account the social context of the client in distress. The social situation emphasized might be the family, the work context, or the treatment context of the person. The social consequences of each intervention also need to be considered. Even accepting a person into therapy is a social act. Being in therapy may define the person as defective and may therefore influence his or her status in the family or at work and is on the record for the future. There are two extreme views of therapy among professionals in the field: One is that therapy is a growth experience that everyone should have; the more therapists are involved with a family the better. The second view is that therapy is for those who have a problem that is handicapping them, that the therapist needs to help them recover as easily and quickly as possible, and that the use of a single therapist avoids the hierarchical conflicts that can occur among multiple therapists.

BRIEF THERAPY

Today brief therapy is fashionable. Its popularity doesn't seem to be based on a concern with outcome but on two other factors: One is the influence of short-term therapists, who since the 1950s particularly with the emergence of behavior therapy and a family-oriented, or social, therapy focused on the present, have attempted to make a paradigm shift in therapy. The other is the role increasingly assumed by systems of managed care in the provision of mental health benefits. Business people who were never trained in therapy and know nothing about it are making the decisions. They say who should do therapy, how it should be done, and for how long. In their naivete they are making a positive renovation of the therapy process. Under their guidance, therapy is becoming more active and directive, and less of an intellectual exercise. Concerned with costs, they expect problems to be clearly formulated and therapy goals to be set; since time is money, they want a quick resolution of symptoms. Teachers of therapy must know how to help trainees set goals and resolve clients' presenting problems. They can no longer merely converse with the trainee and reflect on past influences and traumas in a client's life. They must know what to do and how to teach this to trainees.

WAYS TO TEACH THERAPY

Most therapists first learn about therapy in academia. They are given courses on, and read textbooks about, the different schools of therapy and become experts in ideology. They don't actually do therapy themselves, and it is only on rare occasions that they see videotapes of therapy sessions. As undergraduates, they cannot be given confidential material or attend workshops where such information is made available.

No one can learn to do therapy by reading about it. The first time I taught a class of undergraduates about therapy, I realized how difficult it was to give them any idea of the process when they couldn't do it or see it. They could only read summaries of various approaches. This is like trying to teach someone how to play the violin by having them read what master violinists say about their work. Beginning therapists can do more and more reading and spend longer and longer periods of time in seminars, but ultimately they must go in and do the job. It's only a matter of determining how soon to have them do that.

In this book when I speak of teaching or supervision, I am talking about situations where the trainee has responsibility for a case and is being guided by a supervisor. I find it best to put beginning therapists in the room with clients within the first two or three weeks of their clinical training. The client is protected from errors by the novice because a supervisor is behind the one-way mirror.

There are three basic situations where a supervisor guides a therapist with a case:

1. The teaching supervision of a trainee who is there to learn how to do therapy.
2. The supervision of a colleague who is having difficulty with a particular case and wishes assistance (this might or might not be a teaching supervision).
3. The supervision of a therapist who is learning to be a supervisor (peer supervision is not a teaching situation but primarily a sharing of knowledge).

HOW IS SUPERVISION DONE?

The teaching and learning process of training occurs in three standard ways:

1. A trainee, relying on notes, talks with a supervisor about a case.
2. A trainee plays an audio- or videotape of an interview to a supervisor.
3. The trainee interviews a client in a one-way mirror room or in front of a video camera while being observed by the supervisor, who guides the therapy by telephoning suggestions or bringing the trainee out for discussion.

Conversation Supervision

Talking about a case is the most common form of supervision. It is the cheapest and easiest way to supervise. No equipment is necessary, and the only scheduling issue is when the trainee and supervisor can arrange to have conversations, which add up to hours toward licensing for the trainee.

Therapy, like any art, is taught in an apprenticeship system. The difficulty with conversation supervision is that the participants must collaborate on a case, although neither has seen the other practice the art of psychotherapy. The trainee, under pressure from a client who wants help, must try to describe the situation in a way that enables the supervisor to be helpful. The supervisor listens to this description of the case and wonders what might have happened in the interview to cause the trainee to present the problem this way. The way supervision is conducted is changing, but most supervisors were trained during the nondirective period of therapy and, consequently, wish to avoid telling trainees what to do. Yet this is precisely what many trainees faced with a desperate client want to know. In the past when a trainee asked, "How do I stop this man from beating his wife?" the supervisor was apt to reply, "Let's discuss how upsetting this is to you." This nondirective style of supervising is passing away now, and supervisors are beginning to discuss with their trainees ways to stop the wife beating by clients besides consigning such couples for years to villains and victims groups.

The most serious criticisms of supervisors I've heard recently are that they don't tell the trainees what to do and often don't seem to know what to do themselves, except perhaps to explore the client's problem and its history. I was taken by surprise not long ago by the reaction of a large crowd to a comment I made in an address. I was talking about how therapists might be paid by the cure of a symptom rather than by the hour. I pointed out that this means that therapists would be required to define goals and show specific results in order to get paid. After all, I pointed out, the idea of getting paid by the hour for therapy is an arbitrary decision made by someone in the past. I added, almost in passing, that supervisors might be paid for techniques successfully taught, such as the use of paradox or metaphor, rather than by the hour. A cheer arose from the crowd.

One advantage of conversation supervision is that various kinds of problems can be discussed in relation to the case the trainee is presenting. For example, during the discussion of the troubled marriage of the trainee's client there can be a conversation about similar marital problems and how they were dealt with in therapy.

As with all forms of supervision, the unit under consideration for the supervisor consists of both client and trainee. When the client is not available for observation, the clinical acumen of the supervisor is often directed toward the trainee who is turned into a client. That is, the supervisor, frustrated with trying to determine what must have happened in the clinical interview and hampered by the rule that supervisors shouldn't tell trainees what to do, begins to focus on the trainee's emotional problems and biases. Inasmuch as that endeavor may also become frustrating, the supervisor may end up advising the trainee to go into therapy so he or she won't have further difficulty with clients.

In conversation supervision, the trainee's description is inevitably biased. Not trained to be a participant observer, the trainee tends to provide a portrait of an interview that the supervisor might have perceived quite differently if he or she had been able to actually observe it. When therapy was first observed in one-way mirror rooms in the 1950s, the effect was revolutionary because it became obvious that therapy was not what people said it was. Relationships suddenly became visible, and Harry Stack Sullivan's view that both therapist and client are in the room became self-evident. Before that, the therapist was considered only a blank screen on which the client projected his or her ideas or impulses, and was expected to maintain a neutral stance (the failure of this endeavor being the reprehensible countertransference).

Not only might a trainee therapist censor parts of what happened in a therapy session so as to appear more competent, but a supervisor might collaborate in that misrepresentation. For example, if a therapist and supervisor are committed to a particular approach to therapy, they may implicitly agree to ignore certain issues. I am reminded of a presentation of supposed family therapy by a supervisor and therapist who were interviewing a family in public. As they discussed the way the family members constructed reality, neither supervisor nor therapist mentioned that the adolescent in the family was locked up in a mental hospital and in the interview was asking to be released. The social context was censored from the consultation since the therapy was about inner processes and narratives of the individual and not about actual events in the present.

Conversational supervision can be helpful when a supervisor has previously trained the therapist. The two share an ideology and approach, and the clinical interview under discussion can be described with commonly held concepts and language. The supervisor can think of directives to suggest and can discuss similarities to other cases so that generalizations can be drawn to help the trainee with the next case. Discussing a case and comparing it to similar cases allows for a more general discussion than would result from the time-consuming process of listening to the recorded details of a therapy session.

There are also cases where observation is not essential. For example, a therapist came to a supervisor, who had previously trained her, with the case of a woman who had mysterious physical ailments that incapacitated her. She and her husband seemed to have a marital contract in which she was to have problems and the husband, though exasperated, would take care of her. The therapist's problem was that the husband had written her a letter saying he was in love with her, and in love for the first time in his life. The therapist asked the supervisor what she should do with the letter. Should she show it to the wife or keep it confidential? The supervisor, knowing the competence of this therapist because of her training and, consequently confident of her ability to carry out the proposed actions skillfully, advised her and felt no need to observe her interaction with the client.

Therapy for the Therapist?

If therapy were only a skill, one could teach it as a set of techniques. However, therapists themselves are the instrument through which therapeutic techniques are expressed. And sometimes that instrument has problems. Sometimes the intensity of emotion in a therapeutic session is too much for the therapist to tolerate. Sometimes there is conflict between teacher and trainee. At some time or other, therapists will experience many of the problems that clients do. Often, a therapist is young and at the leaving home stage, which can be distressing. Rather than avoiding disturbing ideas and troubled individuals, as most people do, therapists seek them out every day of their lives. There are personal consequences to work of this sort: As Gregory Bateson once put it, the probe we stick into human beings always has another end that sticks into us.

Sometimes therapists are too anxious to carry out an interview; at other times they compulsively do what isn't helpful to the client. Some therapists are arrogant and can agree with no one, and others have trouble listening. Some cannot stop asking questions and never take a position. When seeing a couple, a therapist can inadvertently side with one partner in a way that prevents change from taking place. Sometimes a therapist feels hopeless and will communicate a hopeless attitude to the client. The supervisor not only has the task of teaching a therapist clinical techniques but also must help the therapist overcome personal difficulties and reach the highest possible level of clinical competence.

Does Personal Therapy Make a Better Therapist?

There is no evidence—and almost no scientific investigation of the issue—that a therapist who has had personal therapy is more successful in treating clients than one who hasn't had therapy. Yet this has been a basic assumption, one that came from the type of training that excluded the experience of observing a therapist at work. It is also an important economic factor in the field of psychotherapy, since a high percentage of clients are therapists-in-training. Not knowing what is actually happening in an interview and worried about what might be, the supervisor can only refer the trainee to personal therapy and prayer.

Of course, there's the argument that a trainee's biases will cause problems in therapy. That might be true. If such a problem occurs with a trainee, the supervisor must solve it. Sending the trainee to therapy is hardly the solution. There's no proof that therapy will change the bias introduced by a therapist's emotional problems. Sigmund Freud suggested that a few months of personal analysis would help trainees become more objective. His remarks have now become the excuse for training analyses in New York lasting an average of seven years. (How could any trainee ever recover from that ideological immersion?) Because personal therapy was accepted as a part of training in the past, it is still required today, even if it is not appropriate for a particular trainee. Family therapy programs run by ex-analysts or psychodynamic therapists usually require family therapy of a trainee. This means that spouses and children must enter therapy whether they like it or not and whether they have problems or not. This is one of several varieties of compulsory therapy and can be considered an improper invasion of the privacy of trainees.

There are merits to personal therapy, and a trainee with problems should certainly seek out that experience. The point here is that it's questionable whether personal therapy makes better therapists in terms of outcome. That conclusion has yet to be proved. When the personal therapy alternative is offered to a trainee, it lets the supervisor off the hook. Rather than help the trainee over a handicap, the supervisor refers the trainee to personal therapy, thus avoiding the task of teaching him or her what to do. If, for example, a trainee is anxious and nervous in an interview, maybe it's because he or she doesn't know what to do; the supervisor should take responsibility for educating the trainee instead of referring the individual for personal therapy. It is in achieving competence that the trainee recovers from the anxiety, not through understanding in personal therapy what makes him or her nervous.

One merit of the therapists' having personal therapy is that they experience feelings of vulnerability and learn what it is like to ask for help. In other words, a therapist can learn empathy for clients by being one.

There are family therapists who don't set clear therapeutic goals or focus on what to do but, instead, emphasize understanding the family system. They put trainees through experiences of sculpting their own families or have them make genograms of their family tree. In various ways they teach trainees what a family system is like by having them explore their own family system. Although an understanding of family systems theory might occur in such a training program, it is never made clear how this knowledge leads to therapy interventions that cause a change in clients. The emphasis is usually on trainees being educated about their own family. What to do with client families isn't emphasized. The implication is that therapists will educate their client families about family systems, just as they themselves were educated.

Traditional personal therapy usually teaches the trainee to focus on the self and is usually individually oriented with an emphasis on self-awareness. It is difficult to train a therapist in a socially oriented active therapy if he or she has had lengthy traditional personal therapy. I find that the more therapy the trainee has had, the more difficult he or she is to train in an active social approach to therapy. Such therapists continue to monitor and analyze themselves even during therapy interviews (e.g., they might ask themselves, "Am I responding to this woman as if she were my mother?"). Sometimes they are so preoccupied with themselves and their own motivations that the client has trouble getting their attention. They also tend to blame the past for problems, as their own therapist did, and to disregard the present context.

Video Supervision:
Observing What Once Happened

Up until the 1950s it was difficult to observe a therapy session because the technical means were not available. To film a session was too expensive to be practical (although occasionally filming was done). I filmed research interviews with families and occasional therapy sessions. The arrival of audiotapes and the reduction in size of recorders made it convenient to record therapy sessions.

By the 1970s it became possible to inexpensively videotape a therapy session. It was immediately apparent that this technology, which made it possible to record and study clinical interviews, would transform training programs in therapy. Critical segments of interviews could be selected and put together in edited teaching tapes. (I recall the business manager of the Philadelphia Child Guidance Clinic at the time protesting our enthusiasm for the new technology by exclaiming, "You're buying those videorecorders like pencils!") Although previously one could observe an interview taking place behind a one-way mirror, being able to see it on videotape, to freeze a frame, and to go back again and again to study a particular segment of the interview gave a new perspective to the nature of therapy, as well as to human interaction in general. Examining the tape in slow motion or fast motion enabled one to see sequences that were not readily apparent at normal speed.

In contrast with conversation supervision, video supervision makes it possible to see therapist and family in action together. Not only is the dialogue and tone of voice preserved, but the body movements and shifting positions of client and therapist are observable and available, once the tape is stopped, for prolonged examination. Often, the way a client sits down provides a wealth of information about his or her relationship with the therapist. (I recall Milton Erickson saying that he was waiting for a woman who had had a significant extramarital or premarital affair not to tell him about it by the way she sat down in the chair.) Such information is hardly available when an interview is merely described from notes.

Although the use of video technology in clinical training can achieve what conversation supervision cannot (enabling the supervisor to see all that was done in the therapy interview and what might have been done), trainees often prefer to describe an interview they conducted rather than present a videotape of it. They feel their inadequacies are exposed and on record. Whether they are uneasy or not, trainees should realize that the benefit of improving their interview skills is so valuable that the discomfort of being observed is worth it. After all, clinical skill is what therapy is about.

As valuable as video technology is for clinical supervision, there are, nevertheless, limitations. The supervisor examining a videotaped interview lacks the opportunity to learn how the client would respond to a new intervention. The supervisor cannot influence past actions. Clinical diagnosis, which is quite different from diagnosis for administrative reasons, occurs when the client responds to what the therapist does. As Salvador Minuchin once put it, "Diagnosis is the way a family moves when you push it."

In summary, supervising by video recordings allows the supervisor to see the therapist in action. The communication exchanged in the session is visible, and its meaning is available. The drawback is that it is too late to change what happened.

Why Be Interested in Body Movement?

Body movement and positioning in the chair, as well as tone of voice, provide the observer with more information than words alone. The metacommunication of the clinical interview, expressed in movement and tone of voice, qualifies whatever is said; only audiovisual recording and live observation provide this information. What is said in a therapeutic conversation can be less important than how it is said in tone and gesture. If a woman says, "I have no complaints about my husband," and touches her nose, she is communicating a different message than if she does not.

Therapy Is Not a Social Occasion

There is a basic premise about therapy that everyone should accept to save much misunderstanding: therapy is not a social context. In a therapy interview, even social comments have a nonsocial significance. The same message means something different in a social context than it does in the therapy interview. (After therapy is over, the therapist and client might meet socially, but during therapy the focus is on change.) For example, in a therapy interview a married couple might turn away from each other or cross their legs away from each other, which can be taken as a statement to the therapist that they are in disagreement. (Of course, such a hypothesis, as with all interpretations of meta messages, should be tentative.) However, if the husband and wife are sitting with friends in a living room and cross their legs away from each other, such body language can have a totally different meaning, or no communicative meaning at all.

Everything said and done in the therapy room should be taken as a message to the therapist about that context. As Gregory Bateson once put it, "Every message is both a report and a command." The report can be about a person's state of mind or situation, but all messages indicate how the other person should respond. In therapy it is the command aspect of messages that is especially important, yet it is often ignored by therapists who only focus on the interior of a person and take what a person says as only a comment about his or her inner nature.

Messages are transmitted not only through a client's words, but also in the way they position themselves in the therapy room. If parents seat a child between them in the room, they are telling the therapist something. If a woman sits so that she is giving a cold shoulder to her husband, that is also a comment to the therapist. In a family interview it is usually best for the therapist to allow family members to sit where they please, thus giving them an opportunity to provide a message by their seating arrangement. (The therapist can always change this arrangement later, if desired.)

Of course, an experienced therapist would never comment on a nonverbal message. Some trainees do this to show how acute they are. Others believe that pointing out clients' body language changes them. However, if the therapist says to a client, "You covered your mouth when you commented on your husband, so you must be concealing something," what can the poor woman do? She can only be angry or confused and uncertain as to how to deal with such rudeness. The therapist might then think of her confusion as a product of deep problems and not as a response to the rudeness. It is best for therapists to assume that clients communicate in different ways, and that when they wish to speak more explicitly about something, they will do so. When body movement is interpreted, the client begins to withhold more and more information for fear the therapist will make upsetting issues explicit. In sum, it is not only disrespectful but a technical error to point out to clients what their indirect communication "really" means.

Why Not Be Sensible and Do Live Supervision?

The most effective way to train a therapist is to use a one-way mirror or a video monitor to observe the trainee actually doing therapy. Coaching a therapist while observing what is happening in the therapy interview is the best way to teach clinical skills. It is the most expensive kind of training, but the cost is much less when trainees are taught in a group. The trainees take turns going into the therapy room to interview the family or individual, while the others watch and learn from observing. The supervisor plans a strategy with the trainee beforehand and telephones suggestions during the interview. The trainee is free to leave the therapy room and consult with the supervisor whenever this is necessary. Such live supervision not only offers trainees the opportunity to observe the use of clinical techniques and to improve their own skills but also protects clients from novice therapists, since the supervisor is available for guidance and intervention at all times.

I believe that live supervision is sufficiently important in the training process that I will discuss it in detail in a later chapter. Here, a few general comments can be made.

The Other Side of the Mirror

In live supervision what happens behind the mirror is as important as what happens in front of it. The behavior behind the mirror, that is, in the training group, will parallel what happens in the therapy room. If the supervisor focuses on the trainee's feelings, he or she will delve into the feelings of clients, and everyone will get in touch with that sort of language.

The hierarchical issues on both sides of the mirror are similar. If a supervisor behaves like an equal or a pal with trainees, the trainees will have difficulty assuming the role of expert in a therapy interview with a family. This is particularly evident when the family has a member out of control. For example, if the therapist wants the parents to be firm with a violent child, the therapist must arrange, directly or indirectly that the parent be firm. For the therapist to do so, the supervisor must arrange that the therapist be firm. The hierarchy in front of the mirror reflects the hierarchy behind it (even in training programs when there is no mirror). Therefore, if the therapy involves a therapist taking charge as the expert in the therapy room, the supervisor must take charge as expert behind the mirror. This does not mean that tyranny is established; it simply means that the supervisor needs to know his or her business when training therapists and the therapist needs to be an expert in helping clients.

In both therapy and supervision, responsibility must be defined. In clinical practice the therapist is responsible for outcome. In live supervision the supervisor is responsible; should the case fail, the supervisor has failed (in peer supervision or the supervision of a colleague with a problem, the same rule does not necessarily apply).

Just as one wishes positive behavior in the therapy room, so too does one wish to have such behavior behind the mirror. When trainees are brought together, it is helpful if the supervisor makes a brief speech about the rules for behavior behind the mirror. The basic rule should be that trainees are not to comment on each other's interviews unless they have a positive suggestion to make. Insightful interpretations, which are usually negative, are not allowed between trainees because they produce bad feeling. What is wanted is high morale. It is appropriate to say, "Perhaps that man would change more quickly if you brought his mother in." It is not helpful to say, "Have you avoided bringing his mother in because you are afraid of mothers?"

Often, supervisees have had previous training in psychodynamic therapy. It is difficult for them to give up making interpretations. They must have help. Part of the problem is that experienced therapists are asked to become students again to learn the brief therapy approach, a position that is awkward for many of them. One therapist, who had been in private practice for a number of years before entering a training program centered on brief therapy, not only differed with his supervisor on ideology and interview techniques, but also found himself with beginners in learning to interview whole families. The supervisor had to deal with the therapist's pride and also had to prevent him from contaminating the discussions with long-term therapy ideas, particularly the notion that one must spend most of a therapy session on the client's past in order to thoroughly understand him or her. The presence of such a trainee can encourage the supervisor to address practical aspects of therapy to educate beginners in the group; the trainee, meanwhile, must be persuaded to learn the principles of brief therapy and to reserve judgment until after he or she observes them in practice.

A supervisor must also prevent trainees from making jokes about, or ridiculing, the clients being observed behind the mirror. Trainees may lose respect for a therapy approach itself if a supervisor condones such comments, which are usually made by trainees who are attempting to gain a sense of superiority for themselves. Competition among trainees should be directed toward the goal of seeing who can be the most kind and competent therapist. It should be clear to the members of a training group that the supervisor is in charge. Ideas and suggestions go to the supervisor and from there to the therapists. That is, when a therapist comes out of the therapy room needing a plan, the group of trainees should not behave like a democratic group and bombard him or her with ideas. Instead, the supervisor should communicate with the trainee. If the supervisor opens up the discussion so that everyone can contribute, the comments and suggestions from the other trainees are organized by the supervisor.

There are teaching approaches in which the training group is reflective and democratic and no one is responsible for failure. This approach is, essentially, peer supervision. There are also those who argue that training should involve cotherapy, with the teacher being in the room with the trainee rather than behind the mirror. Others argue that because ultimately the trainee must face a client alone, why not begin doing that?

Supervisors must choose what kind of group they want for a training atmosphere. Members of a training group work better together if there are no regular nonparticipant observers (although occasional guests should be welcome); that is, all members should have to expose themselves by doing therapy in front of the group. Observers who do not do therapy but only watch others tend to become critical and even supercilious; they imply that they could do better, but they never have to demonstrate their expertise. If all members of the training group must participate in doing the therapy, they tend to work together and to help each other.

SHOULD EVERYTHING BE SHARED
WITH THE CLIENTS?

Since the time of ancient Egypt the healer, or shaman, has had to grapple with the issue of whether to share ideas with the people they treat or maintain an aura of mystery. Magic works best without sharing its premise, but what about therapy? Should therapists share their strategies with clients? A supervisor must choose what kind of boundary will be drawn around the therapy group. For example, he or she may decide that the therapists-in-training should keep their deliberations private, outside the hearing of the client, and should consider the ideas and procedures planned to be the business of the therapist, not the client. Should clients insist on knowing the rationale for the therapy approach or for a particular intervention, the therapist can state it. However, ordinarily the therapist's strategies and premises are not imposed on the client unless the therapist has reason to believe that such an approach would facilitate change.

In this egalitarian age there are supervisors in this country who argue that therapy should be collaborative. They even argue that family therapists should not be authoritative and impose their ideas on clients but should take a vote with family members on issues. Suppose one wishes to have a mother with a problem son keep a log of his good and bad behavior for a week. The supervisor might have as a goal that the mother will respond differently to the son. Instead of becoming angry, she would make a note and would therefore be responding in unexpected ways as far as the son is concerned. Should the therapist share the idea of this plan with the mother? One could discuss the purpose of the plan with her, and she would probably still do it. But if the possibility exists that she will feel criticized or refuse to participate, what has the therapist gained by democratically sharing the therapy plan with her? The therapist has only responded to an ideological position, not to the mother.

It can be argued that a therapist needs to be particularly careful about sharing certain premises with a family. Let us say, for example, that a therapist has hypothesized that an adolescent boy attempted suicide as a way of helping his parents stabilize their marriage. The therapist might be tempted to share that idea with the parents to emphasize the positive motives of the adolescent, but no couple wants to hear that they are in such bad shape that their child feels he must sacrifice his life for them. If it is true that he attempted suicide to help his parents, the parents would be upset and angry at him and at each other. He would have increased his self-destructive behavior. The therapist would defeat therapy by sharing a therapeutic hypothesis. If the hypothesis is wrong and he was attempting suicide not to help his parents but for other reasons, the therapist would be revealing a serious error. Supervisors should avoid putting their trainees in no-win situations with their clients.

The supervisor must also decide whether to meet a trainee's client who wishes to meet the person behind the mirror. Again, it is a question of whether or not to share the machinery of therapy with the client. Sometimes the therapist can respond by saying that when the client's problem is resolved, he or she can then meet the supervisor. By that time, clients usually don't care whether they do or not.

What is suggested here is that supervisors and trainees think through practices that have been carried over from the past and that might no longer be useful. For example, suppose a client asks a therapist, "Are you married?" What should the supervisor advise the trainee to answer? A traditionally trained supervisor would advise the therapist to say, "I wonder why you ask me that." Today we should realize that such a response is from the period when the theorists considered the therapist to be a blank screen on which the client projected ideas and impulses. Clients were thought to be manipulative, or behaving inappropriately, when they asked for practical information about the therapist. The emphasis was on the client's fantasies, not the real world. Today most therapists believe that clients have a right to know if their therapist is married or has children. The therapist who feels there is a hidden agenda behind such a question can reply, "Yes, I'm married. Why do you ask?" In that way the therapist can be human and also deal with different aspects of the question. In this time of change in therapy, various kinds of behavior in therapists and clients must be reconsidered. Apparently, with the development of family therapy, therapists become more human in their responses, a development that has spread to therapies based on other ideologies.

VARIATIONS IN THE CONCEPT OF SUPERVISION

There are cultural differences in training as in therapy. Family therapy was born in the United States, and many of the procedures are typically

American. Milton Erickson, who had a great influence on new developments in therapy, typically gave examples from rural American life.
Individual therapy, with its origins in Europe, emphasized the ideas of
early psychologists. One could not expect Freud to discuss ways of
persuading a cow to leave a barn, as Erickson did. With the shift to
family-oriented therapy the real world entered the therapy room, and
fantasies and philosophy became less of a focus.

The idea of a group of therapists behind the mirror is also an
American approach. The notion of a leader who draws on the ideas of
followers but makes the final decision and takes responsibility for what
happens reflects the typical American emphasis on individualism. This
can be contrasted with the approach of family therapists in Japan, where,
as I understand it, the supervisor and the training group behind the
mirror must reach a consensus on what is to be done; the supervisor then
is essentially a representative of the group.

There is, of course, the possibility that a supervisor who takes
responsibility as an expert will become a tyrant with his or her trainees
and will expect them to mimic his or her clinical ideas and behavior.
There is some justification for concern about this possibility. There are
arrogant supervisors out in the world who don't encourage independent
thought in their trainees but simply put them down and expect them to
adopt the views they present to them. This risk exists in part because
therapy is learned in an apprenticeship process. Ideally, one apprentices
oneself to an expert, learns what he or she has to teach, and then
develops one's own individual approach, but there are apprentice-thera-
pists who never go beyond what they were taught by their supervisor.
Others develop a solid base of skill and knowledge and generate new
ideas. The goal of supervision is to produce therapists who improve upon
what they learn.

This particular way of thinking about live supervision is one among
many. There are those who argue that supervision (as well as therapy)
should be less hierarchical and more collaborative. They prefer a team
approach without a supervisor as leader, and sometimes they like to have
the team sit with the family rather than behind a mirror. There are also
therapists who argue that training should include the use of cotherapy,
with the trainee being in the room with the client as the teacher conducts
the therapy.

I do not recommend these approaches here. I am concerned that
supervisors who use these approaches may do so because they're reluctant to take responsibility for what happens in therapy. Sharing responsibility with a team, with clients themselves, or with a cotherapist is a way
to avoid it. I believe that the supervisor needs ideas from the group of
therapists behind the mirror but that he or she needs to take responsibil-

ity for what happens to the client. I am also concerned that many supervisors may not know what to teach a trainee to do about a particular problem and that sharing with a team the task of devising a plan to resolve the problem avoids having to know what to do. Conversation replaces action in training and in therapy.

I believe that using cotherapy in training only teaches the trainee to sit back and watch the teacher work. Since the student ultimately has to take responsibility for treating clients, why not begin with the trainee doing the therapy and the supervisor observing its progress from behind the mirror?

2
THE SUPERVISOR

SELECTING A SUPERVISOR

It is ideal if a supervisor is older, mature, wise, and experienced in life as well as in doing therapy. The wiser the supervisor is the more patience he or she is likely to have and the more training will benefit. Of course, trainees typically do not have the ideal supervisor, but a discussion of the characteristics of such an individual can be helpful. It is the wiser trainee who learns whatever he or she can from each teacher, even from an inadequate supervisor. It is even a wiser trainee who will relocate to spend a period of time with the best supervisor available. If one is planning to devote a lifetime to doing therapy, a year or two at the learning stage is not a great sacrifice.

It is best if one's supervisor has been married and has had children, meaning that he or she is familiar with the ordinary vicissitudes of life, in addition to being experienced in conducting therapy. Moreover, time on the therapy side of the mirror helps provide empathy for everyone involved. The supervisor should be a kindly person because of the difficulties and distress that must be dealt with on both sides of the mirror. He or she should also be ambitious, conscientious, and determined to achieve success with every therapy case.

Being a good therapist does not guarantee that one will become a good supervisor. Sometimes administrators who admire the skill of a therapist wish to elevate him or her to a supervisory position in the belief that one ability is relevant to the other. However, therapist and supervisor require different skills. Therapists must think on their feet (or seat) in the middle of therapy action; in contrast, a supervisor behind the mirror has the time to be reflective and the opportunity to see the wider picture without being forced into an immediate response.

When I was in private practice, I sometimes had difficulty thinking of a directive in the emotional action of the first interview. I had trouble being objective. Sometimes I'd tell clients that I wanted them to come back in a week and I would give them a helpful directive at that time. I would say this without knowing what the directive would be, but I was confident that in a week I'd think of one. Other therapists can easily think of what to do within the interview. One of the reasons I turned to supervision was because I welcomed the opportunity to be more distant from the data and therefore more objective.

The teaching supervisor must respond not only to what happens in the therapy room but also to what happens with the training group behind the mirror. The unit of observation is both the trainee group and the therapy interview. A supervisor who is focused on the therapy situation may neglect the training mandate and vice versa.

Some therapists who are enthusiastic about doing therapy have problems when they become supervisors. They are bored behind the mirror and would like to be in the therapy room, where the action is. There are also supervisors who gather their clinical data by interacting with clients and observing their responses. They have trouble acquiring information by observing clients through a one-way mirror. Therefore, they enter the therapy room to "help" the therapist, sometimes creating a theory to rationalize why that is a good way to supervise. I recommend that the supervisor stay behind the mirror. Too often, therapists have trouble regaining status after the supervisor enters the therapy room and takes charge. This is particularly so if the supervisor proves to be difficult or incompetent. Trainees also learn to take more responsibility if it is established at the outset that the supervisor will not be coming into the therapy room to rescue them.

If one is an administrator hiring a supervisor, the emphasis should be on the issues outlined here. If one is a trainee selecting a supervisor, one should be concerned not only with how wise and worthy of respect the individual is but also with how well one gets along with him or her. After all, supervisor and trainee will spend many hours together struggling with highly charged and upsetting emotional situations.

THE GOALS OF TRAINING

Training can be thought of as occurring in stages. Besides the acquisition of the general knowledge required to be a professional, the specific goal in therapy training is achieving competence in interviewing. Whether it is thought of as a humanistic interchange or a technical skill, therapy is essentially interview technique. Trainees need to be able to skillfully interview individuals, couples, and families. They should be able to deal well with children, adolescents, adults, and the elderly. They should interview in such a way that problems are clarified, solutions are emphasized, and positive destinations have become clear. Trainees need to approach an interview with a sense of opportunity rather than trepidation. That is, a trainee stopped in the hall of the therapy center and asked to see a family that just walked in should be able to confidently reply, "Sure," rather than anxiously ask, "What sort of family?"

In the second stage—and this can require a second year of training—the trainee must become skillful in using a variety of interventions and know which ones to use in a given situation. For example, the trainee might be capable of solving a problem quickly with a client or family who has struggled with the problem for a long time but should also be aware of the fact that a quick success might make him or her too powerful in relation to the client. In other words, trainees must learn to anticipate clients' reactions to interventions, even successful ones. Therapists want to avoid having the client or family relapse out of a need to unbalance the power. Supervisors must teach therapists at least two ways to prevent relapse: (1) by encouraging a relapse so skillfully that the family or client overcomes the therapist's power by not relapsing, in which case everyone wins, or (2) by avoiding getting credit for a positive change (if it is a mystery to the therapist why the change has taken place, then he or she is not made responsible for it by the client or family). The second stage is completed when trainee therapists can do what they have been taught to do by their supervisor.

Finally, it must be acknowledged that if trainees can only do what their supervisors can do, the training is not fully successful. If supervisors produce graduating trainees who think and act just like them, success is limited. The art of teaching includes the goal of encouraging trainees to create and test new and original procedures. Toward the end of training supervisors should be pleasantly surprised by the novel interventions their trainees make, interventions which the supervisor has not thought of. The most difficult aspect of training is teaching the art of innovation, which is necessary because clients and their problems change and new approaches must be developed.

I think it might be questioned whether past generations of supervisors have indeed produced therapists who are more innovative than they are. Have the followers of the teachers of the different therapy approaches, particularly the family therapies, made a comparable or superior contribution? If they have done no better than their teachers, is it not the fault of the teachers? Of course, most innovators in a field, especially in the field of therapy, have an orthodoxy against which to clarify their ideas. Their followers do not have that opportunity and can inherit confusion.

There are, of course, many goals of training. Therapists must learn how to become involved with a client and also how to disengage at the appropriate time. Supervisors can encourage these skills during training, but ultimately therapists must acquire them on their own. Therapists must also develop skill in two kinds of interviewing: (1) conversing with a client in such a way that a climate for change is established and (2) making an intervention that will bring about a change.

A therapist must learn how to systematically conduct an interview, and this takes both knowledge and practice. When I began to do therapy, I realized that I didn't know how to conduct a therapeutic interview. Although I searched the literature, I found little guidance. The only guide I could find was *The Psychiatric Interview*[1] by Harry Stack Sullivan. Years later, when I was training a number of therapists, I wrote a text, *Problem-Solving Therapy: New Strategies for Effective Family Therapy,*[2] which included information on how to conduct a first interview. (My own experience had taught me that the beginning therapist needs help in just learning how to say hello and who to say that to.)

There's a danger that therapists will ultimately return to old ways of doing therapy after they finish their training. During training they learn to do innovative, brief therapy and to avoid procedures that make therapy more difficult. To maintain their expertise it is important that they get work in a context where the therapy of their training is appropriate. Unfortunately, that's not always possible. As we know, one's social context largely determines what one thinks. Therapists who work in a context where innovative and brief therapy is not appropriate will have to respond to that reality. They might, for example, be able to find employment only in an inpatient unit. They must work and think in a way that is appropriate to clients in custody. (Such an extreme circumstance might be unusual, but every therapy context, including private practice, determines how the therapist will work. It might not be in ways the person was trained in the more flexible training setting.) For example, years ago I was developing a family-oriented brief therapy and spent some time with hospitalized patients and their families. I concluded that it is pointless to do any therapy at all until a discharge date is set, for I discovered that when the problem person is hospitalized, the rest of the family just says the right things. However, when their therapist says,

---

[1]Sullivan, H. S. (1970). *The psychiatric interview.* New York: Norton.

[2]Haley, J. (1987). *Problem-solving therapy: New strategies for effective family therapy* (2nd ed.). San Francisco: Jossey-Bass.

"Your son is being discharged next Monday morning," families respond with more motivation and interest in what happens in the real world.

WHAT TO TELL A TRAINING GROUP

It might be helpful to provide a detailed guideline to be given to a beginning group of trainees including what they are expected to do. It is assumed the trainees are therapists with experience, not still in graduate school.

1. Trainees will take turns planning a therapy session with the supervisor before entering the interview room behind the mirror to begin the therapy.

2. There are seminars on topics relevant to the cases being seen. Trainees will learn how to introduce to clients the one-way mirror or camera and the release forms that must be signed. Classes can simulate a family therapy session so that trainees can practice these introductions (role playing is performed for this purpose only and not to practice interviewing or making interventions).

3. The students are advised that whatever their background in therapy, they will be taught a particular approach in this training. After learning it, they can then decide whether or not to continue it in their work setting.

4. No psychodynamic interpretations are allowed. Competition about who sees the most awful aspects of a client or family will be prevented; trainees must emphasize the positive in whatever comments they make. They must share the knowledge they have gained from their unique backgrounds in ways that are positive.

5. The supervisor is in charge behind the mirror and is responsible for the outcome of the therapy. The group speaks through the supervisor to the trainee conducting the therapy and does not bombard him or her with ideas from everyone during an interview discussion.

6. When the supervisor makes a suggestion on the telephone during the therapy, it is a suggestion, not an order. The trainee might have a different opinion and should state that. There are times, however, when the supervisor will convey an order to the trainee, since it is the supervisor who is responsible for the success or failure of the case. If the trainee objects to the directive the supervisor has conveyed over the telephone, he or she should leave the therapy room and consult with the supervisor to reach agreement on how to proceed.

7. Trainees must expect to do a kind of therapy they have not previously done and to intervene in ways that enlarge their clinical

repertoire. However, they should not do what is against their principles but should negotiate with the supervisor until agreement is reached.

8. When the telephone in the therapy room lights up, the trainee should pick it up, listen, hang up, and go on with the interview. There should not be an exaggerated response to the call. The supervisor uses the telephone primarily to make suggestions in line with a previously determined plan; therefore, the calls should be brief and to the point. A major intervention, such as an ordeal strategy, should not originate on the telephone but should be discussed behind the mirror.

9. The ultimate goal of training is to enable therapists to not need the supervisor and to succeed with cases because of the special knowledge gained in the training. Likewise, the goal of therapy is to enable the client to become independent of the therapist as quickly as possible.

10. A follow-up interview with a client or family in the one-way mirror room a few months after therapy is often helpful. The family is asked about what happened in their therapy and what they think caused a change. Their response often surprises trainees because the intervention they assumed to cause change might not be the one the family identifies as such. The follow-up interview has another effect: It increases a trainee's commitment to a case by reminding him or her that the client or family might be called back to report to the group on their experience with therapy.

WHO IS MANAGING THE CARE?

Most therapists were trained in a period when therapy could be a long and leisurely process. the focus was on reflection about the past and the nature of problems in the present. There was no pressure on the therapist to induce a rapid change. Young people today can hardly believe that long-term therapy was once accepted. I recall doing in the 1950s a brief therapy using hypnosis and family therapy and dealing with symptoms as communicative phenomena. When I lectured on resolving a symptom quickly, the audience of therapists thought it was improper, if not immoral, to do therapy that lasted only a few session. They were accustomed to advising a client not to expect a change in less than a year, and a therapy of several years was common. Clients expected little from therapists in those days, and so there was no pressure for change. Clients did not expect the therapist to focus on a problem, and it was argued that brief therapy must be shallow. Therapists needed relatively few clients, since they were seen for a long time. How therapy was financed affected the length of therapy as it does today.

Over the years there was a slow acceptance of brief therapy, with both clients and therapists increasingly likely to expect therapy to be short-term. This meant that therapists needed to be trained to be directive and active. Where could one find such supervisors? I can recall commuting from San Francisco to Phoenix to get supervision from Milton Erickson because he was the only therapist I knew (and I had researched a number of therapists as part of Bateson's research project) who used brief therapy. The referrals for a brief therapy practice in those days were often people who had failed in years of long-term therapy. There were also referrals from physicians who did not think it should take years to cure a patient of a symptom like a phobia and who would therefore refer their patients for hypnotherapy. (Perhaps I should add that even though the goal was to make the therapy brief, this was not always achieved. I recall once doing "brief therapy" for 3 years with a client I could not cure or dismiss.)

Today the financing of therapy is being transformed, and therapists must learn to conduct short-term, symptom-focused therapy. The insurance people are deciding what therapy should be, how long it should last, and who should do it. The debates among therapists about how therapy should be done are being superseded by profit-and-loss concerns, even more than in the past. Therapists today attempt to become chosen providers rather than rely on the traditional referral process. Supervisors who were not trained in brief therapy are being required to teach such an approach since that is the kind that fits the limits imposed by the insurance companies. This book presents a short-term therapy approach that was developed many years before managed care emerged.

An important task for therapists today is to maintain the integrity of therapy and to avoid compromising their beliefs just to satisfy a group of business people who don't know what therapy is or what it could be. The danger to the therapy field is that those people with financial control will encourage inadequate treatment by therapists who have the least training and charge the lowest fees. If therapy is done improperly and fails, the reputations of all therapists will suffer. On the other hand, insurance companies are having the positive effect of focusing therapists on the psychological problems people want to resolve and on their desire to get over those problems as quickly as possible.

Let us hope that therapists of different schools and opposing factions will come together to maintain an ethical position in this time of change. Each therapist and each supervisor needs to take an ethical position and to stand firm in their insistence with managed care people on how therapy should be done with a case and for what length of time. Fortunately, it seems that progress is being made in convincing these people that the cheapest therapist is rarely the most effective in the long run.

INTERVENTION FOLLOWS SUPERVISION

Teaching therapists means giving them an expanding knowledge of human capabilities. Teaching them a range of interview skills to solve their clients' difficulties, and helping them overcome personal problems that interfere with their ability to conduct therapy effectively, is part of the task. It has become evident that how one does therapy and how one teaches a trainee to do therapy are synonymous. If the supervisor does insight therapy, he or she will teach by providing the trainee with personal insight. If one does a directive, brief therapy, one directs the trainee in what to do. It can be confusing to trainees if the supervisor teaches a theory appropriate to long-term insight therapy while supposedly guiding them in brief therapy techniques. As therapy changes, supervision must change. Because the field is now in transition, marked by a confusing mixture of past and present ideas, therapy and supervision can conflict with each other.

If a therapist explores and interprets unconscious ideas and emotions to a client in therapy, one can assume that his or her supervisor is exploring the unconscious ideas and emotions of the therapist. If the supervisor asks the therapist to create a genogram family tree or asks for an extensive social history from him or her, the therapist will discuss the past with his or her clients. If a therapist focuses on the client's presenting problem, his or her supervisor will be focusing on the specific strengths and weaknesses of the therapist. What happens in the therapy room is formally the same as what happens in the supervisory room.

THE PSYCHODYNAMICS OF TRAINING: PAST AND PRESENT

In the psychodynamic period, therapy and training were so well coordinated that they seemed to merge into a single process. The set of ideas might seem old-fashioned today, but they are still used by many teachers since that is how they were trained. Here are some of the features that characterized the psychodynamic approach:

1. Psychotherapy was thought of as a medical specialty, with a medical degree being required for the highest prestige as a therapist. As a result, words like *health*, *treatment*, and *patient* were imposed.
2. The focus was on the individual, and no families were seen in training or in therapy. Therapists did not speak to the relatives of their

patients. The family was considered a negative influence that somehow caused patients to become what they were.

3. No directives were given to patients or trainees. Nor did the therapist initiate what was to happen in therapy or in training. The psychodynamic therapist was a responder, not an initiator.

4. With both clients and trainees, the emphasis was on applying the same approach to all. There were no changes in the approach for different classes, ethnic groups, or kinds of people.

5. Patients were taught the theory of the therapy or were encouraged to read about it, so the ideas became part of the popular culture.

6. The focus was on the interior of the trainee or the client. The unconscious was defined by the theory of repression as a place full of unfortunate impulses and negative desires. It was not to be trusted. A therapist would not tell a client or trainee to follow their impulses. (After all, what might they do?)

7. Symptoms were considered to be maladaptive and inappropriate, carried over from the past, with no present social function. In therapy the truth about the influence of the past was sought, not a hypothesis about the patient's present problem.

8. Therapy consisted of bringing about insight into unconscious motivations and tracing ideas to their origins in the past. The present was considered secondary gain and not primary. It was thought that ideas caused a person's social behavior and that they needed to be changed. It was not assumed that ideas were a result of a relationship.

9. Personal therapy was the primary basis of training. The assumption was that a therapist whose emotional problems were resolved would automatically know how to solve the problems of others. Trainees learned how to do therapy by observing their own.

These characteristics of psychodynamic training and treatment are sufficient to make it clear that therapy and training were synonymous. Most supervisors of therapy today were trained in that approach or in some modification of it and are being asked to abandon those ideas. Today many supervisors are attempting to teach a new form of therapy based on premises that are exactly the opposite of those on which their own training was based. Let us review some of the changes all of us are adapting to, whether as trainee or supervisor:

1. Therapy is no longer considered a medical specialty, and many therapists are avoiding the use of such words as *sickness*, *health*, and *patient* for clients in therapy. Psychiatry has less influence over the practice of psychotherapy. Anyone who has trained psychiatric residents over the years has seen a steady decrease in their training in therapy. Once among the best trained, many psychiatry departments today do not

emphasize training in therapy. As psychiatry becomes more biologically based and confined to psychopharmacology, residents are given less opportunity to learn therapy skills. There are psychiatry departments where therapy is an elective. Nor do psychiatrists often attend workshops on psychotherapy. More preoccupied with exploring the complexities of medication, many psychiatrists do not learn how to do talk therapy; consequently, they insist that medication, rather than therapy, be used for psychological problems. When therapists wish medication to be reduced or discontinued because it is incapacitating their client, they often find it difficult to communicate with the psychiatrist involved. Sometimes a supervisor must negotiate for them.

2. For many years it has been common for family therapists to not only speak to their client's relatives but to invite them into therapy. The family isn't considered a negative force but a resource for bringing about change. As part of the change in ideology, symptoms are now considered not maladaptive but appropriate behavior in the client's social situation, and it is the social situation, such as the family or work group, that has to change in order to resolve the client's symptom. With this view, it is logical to focus therapy on the present situation, not the past. When a therapist proposes a social function for a symptom, it need not be a true one but, rather, one that guides the therapist in what to do. For example, a therapist may hypothesize that an adolescent is misbehaving to stabilize his family. That idea can guide the therapist to action even if a research investigation might not find support for it. We are dealing with hypotheses, not truths, and with all the consequences of that.

3. Most brief therapies require that the therapist give directives to bring about change. Action must occur. It is assumed that behavior brings about ideas in response to the social situation, not that ideas cause behavior. It is not assumed that insight causes change but, rather, that change can cause insight. Therefore, the focus is on directives for new behavior, not on interpretations. The client's narratives, or fantasies, change as his or her relationships with others change, not vice versa.

4. There have always been two views of the unconscious: (1) that it is a repository of negative ideas and (2) that it is a positive force that guides people to what is best for them. This was the view of hypnosis adopted by many hypnotists, including Milton Erickson. In contemporary therapy the focus is on what is positive in the life, or the unconscious, of the client, since that can be encouraged and can lead to positive change. People are taught to trust their unconscious. A supervisor can even say to a trainee therapist, "Follow your impulses in the session." It is now considered the job of the supervisor to get trainees over personal difficulties that interfere with their therapy. Referring them out for personal therapy is not done unless a supervisor does not know what else to do. As therapy changes, supervisors find themselves taking responsibility

for training effective therapists by helping their trainees overcome personal handicaps is an important focus of supervisory training.

5. Most contemporary therapists do not apply the same therapy method to all clients. They change their approach with the problem and the client. That is one reason why it is difficult to describe the new brief therapy approach. The therapist is taught to devise a unique therapy for each case. This is difficult to teach and to learn. Everyone finds it easier to find a method that can be used with everybody.

A problem afflicting the field now is the antitherapeutic diagnostic system. Supervisors need to teach therapists about the problems of clients in a diagnostic language that guides the therapist in what to do. For example, saying that a child who won't go to school has a "school phobia" isn't a helpful way for a supervisor to describe the child. To diagnose him as having a "school avoidance" problem is sensible since it suggests what might be done—prevent the child from avoiding school.

NEW WAYS OF TRAINING

When we turn to the question of how to help therapists get over personal difficulties that cause a problem with clients, the similarity between the training relationship and the therapy relationship suggests an obvious plan: Supervisors can adapt all the innovative techniques of therapy being developed today for use in helping trainee therapists.

Some supervisors think of a trainee's ineffectiveness in terms of underlying emotional problems—a view from past generations—rather than a lack of skill or a response to an inhibiting diagnosis and social context. For example, a supervisor might check first whether a trainee in trouble is caught between a case supervisor and an academic supervisor who are teaching opposite views. Trainees can become paralyzed when responding to conflicting authorities, just as clients can who are caught in conflictual relationships in their families. If teachers are focused on the interior of their trainees, the trainees external situation is ignored. Such supervisors have a world of new discoveries to make if they shift to a social view of problems.

The problems of the trainee can be resolved by changes in relation to the supervisor, just as the client's problems can be resolved in relation to the therapist. The techniques of brief therapy are available to the therapy teacher: He or she can use a problem-solving orientation, or a solution emphasis, or a narrative approach; or restrain a trainee from change with the use of a paradox or metaphors; or offer an ordeal, or use straightforward advice and directives. Supervisors can be active and directive, just as therapists today are. If a trainee has a problem and "cannot help it," the supervisor can use indirect techniques, as does the therapist with a client who "cannot help it."

ERICKSON AS SUPERVISOR

Milton Erickson is a classic example of a teacher who used similar approaches with trainees and clients. Let me give a brief description of what he did with me over the years, although what he did was complex and deserves more extended discussion.

I went into practice many years ago as a hypnotherapist and family therapist. I learned hypnosis from Erickson at a seminar in 1953. John Weakland and I conducted hypnotic evenings where anyone interested could come and have some experience with hypnosis. For several years I taught hypnosis to psychologists and psychiatrists in Palo Alto who wanted seminars on the subject, particularly in connection with brief therapy. Although many of them liked hypnotherapy, they didn't want to use it themselves, and began to refer patients to me. When I went into practice, I discovered that I knew how to hypnotize people by means of a whole range of inductions but that I had no idea how to use hypnosis to change them. Hypnosis has at least three major applications: (1) the individual experience of a trance, as in meditation; (2) the research application where parameters such as the limits and depth of a trance are investigated; and (3) the clinical use of trance, where one hypnotizes someone to change them. Before I consulted with Erickson, I realized that with all my experience I only knew the personal and research applications of hypnosis. How to use hypnosis to change someone was quite a different endeavor. That's when I began to consult with Erickson about my cases.

I had been doing research on therapy for some time, with Erickson as one of the subjects, and I knew his unusual skills as a hypnotist. At that time hypnosis was taught to therapists only through weekend seminars by Erickson and others. Freud had turned against hypnosis, and he had the power to prevent it from being taught. It was not easy to find a hypnosis consultant, and I was fortunate to have studied the hypnosis approach of Erickson. I also realized that he had a special therapy approach that was brief and directive. I began to consult with him about cases in my practice; I wrote up many of these discussions in *Conversations with Erickson*.[3] I visited him for a week once a year for many years. My problem when I began was not that I wasn't successful with my clients. I was changing clients, but I didn't know how. Therefore, I wasn't

[3]Haley, J. (1985). *Conversations with Erickson* (3 vols.). New York: Norton.

sure I could repeat my successes. When I went to talk with Erickson, I learned to give a name to some of the things I was doing. For example, I had cured a woman of severe headaches but didn't know how I had done it. Talking with Erickson, I realized that I had been scheduling and encouraging her headaches, and that could be considered a paradoxical technique. Over the years, Erickson had great influence on my therapeutic technique and on my teaching of therapy.

Here are a few of the premises Erickson taught me: In all his supervisory conversations, Erickson taught that people were changeable and curable. Even the most difficult person could be changed. I recall him saying of a woman he had been struggling to change for some time, with determined anger in his voice, "That woman is still defeating me." There was no question in his mind that the therapist's job is to change people and that failure is the fault of the therapist. He rarely referred cases out to others; the buck stopped with him. He occasionally reported on a case on which he gave up. I recall the case of a young boy that Erickson referred out because, as he told the boy, he could not succeed with him because he got under his skin. This was rare for Erickson. He did not blame the boy but took responsibility for the treatment failure himself. It is Erickson's attitude that leads me to say to supervisees, "I want you to continue with this client until there's a cure or until you turn 80 years old, whichever comes first." Often clients change when they believe the therapist will never give up.

Erickson taught that one should be directive at a time when only nondirective therapy was proper. He taught the use of directives by telling case metaphors and by using hypnosis. All of his cases illustrate a way of taking action to influence and change a client or a trainee. He did not categorize his directives, but a considerable range is evident in his case anecdotes. He would use straightforward directives: He told clients what to do, sometimes insisting on major changes in living. He also offered advice, coached clients to achieve something they wished, and used ordeals that helped people abandon a symptom.

Erickson could also do nothing. I recall him demonstrating hypnosis before a large audience: He asked for a volunteer to come up so that he could demonstrate resistance. A young man came forward and stood in front of him. Although Erickson just stood there, I saw the young man go into a trance. Later I asked Erickson what he did to put that young man in a trance. He said he didn't do anything. "But he went into a trance," I insisted. "You must have done something." Erickson said, "No, I did not." He added, "That young man came up in front of all those people. I wasn't doing anything, and somebody had to do something, so he went into a trance." I'm sure that with trainees Erickson would at times do nothing, thus forcing the trainee to act.

Let me give an example of a straightforward directive Erickson offered me when I asked him what to do with a case. I was seeing a couple, and the wife complained of a problem that was driving her to distraction: On Saturday mornings she would vacuum all the rooms in the house, and her husband would follow her from room to room and watch her. This made her nervous and she asked him to stop. When he continued this behavior, she asked me how to stop him. I offered a few practical suggestions, but her husband did not change. I asked Erickson—who always had a solution, as a good supervisor should—what he would do with this problem. He suggested that the woman vacuum the rooms as usual the following Saturday, that she permit her husband to follow her from room to room. After vacuuming she was to carry the vacuum bag full of dirt and dust from room to room and make a pile of dust on the floor in each room. When she finished, she was to say, "Well, that is done," and she was to leave the dirt in piles until the next Saturday. When I asked Erickson why this would work, he said, "It's obvious." Pressed for an explanation, he said that human beings cannot tolerate absurdity, that if the wife cleans and then makes a mess where she has cleaned, the husband will not be able to tolerate the situation and will leave the field. I gave the wife the task, and the husband stopped following her from room to room.

Erickson would give a straight directive when advising a therapist about a case but it was more common for him to listen to a description of a case and then talk about a similar case he had had. His case descriptions were like metaphors that taught one how to think about an issue. His metaphors would suggest not only what to do with a particular client but also stimulate one's own imagination to create new interventions.

Erickson would also give suggestions that were indirect and that had a delayed effect on both trainees and clients. I recall talking with him about a woman I was treating who had phantom limb pain. She had lost an arm to cancer, and she continued to feel it in pain. I hypnotized her with arm levitation of her phantom limb—she pointed to it as it lifted. I thought this was a rather unique hypnotic induction and might deserve a paper. I told Erickson about it, but he was unresponsive and talked about other things. A day or two later he discussed a case of pain with me, saying that one should not induce a trance in a painful area but in a more positive place. After that session I found myself thinking that perhaps I should not have induced a trance focusing on my client's painful arm. I learned the lesson more thoroughly because I arrived at the conclusion myself.

With both clients and trainees Erickson used hypnosis, and in both situations the person might or might not know it was happening. His primary teaching process was trance. I think at times he hypnotized whomever he was talking with as a way to keep from being bored. He was constantly experimenting with different forms of influence, either with clients or trainees. With both, he seemed to often arrange amnesia; one was always a bit uncertain of what one had learned—or whether one had learned anything—because there was time lost in conversations with him.

TYPES OF HYPNOSIS

Most forms of therapy have their origins in hypnosis. The psychodynamic school began with hypnosis, and the learning theory schools are based on the contributions of Pavlov, who was a hypnotist. Family therapy approaches, too, had practitioners trained in hypnosis. A part of the breakdown of orthodoxy in the 1950s was the acceptance of hypnosis by the American Medical Association, paving the way for psychiatrists and other doctors to be taught this art. Now the largest meetings on therapy of any kind are given by the Milton H. Erickson Foundation, and the foundation also trains many therapists.

Even people who do not practice direct hypnosis can use training in hypnosis-inducing skills. One learns how to join a client most effectively, just as one learns to give directives. Hypnosis training teaches the use of metaphors in messages as well as straightforward directives. Besides the use of hypnosis in emergencies, there are various symptoms for which hypnosis can be more effective than conversational approaches.

The problem for therapists is finding out how to get training in clinical hypnosis. There are at least three kinds of hypnotic training: One can learn self-hypnosis for a variety of purposes. One can learn to hypnotize people for research purposes to investigate the capabilities of trance behavior. Neither of these approaches is particularly relevant to clinical hypnosis, where a therapist attempts to relieve a person of a problem. To learn clinical hypnosis one must watch a teacher hypnotize; one is then watched by the teacher, who can guide one's actions. This is how hypnosis was taught in the 19th century. This requires a setting where there are clients to practice on. A seminar in which therapists hypnotize each other can teach participants how to induce a trance, but it does not teach them how to change people. That can only be done in practice. If a supervisor doesn't wish to practice hypnosis with clients or to demonstrate it, another alternative is for the supervisor to remain behind the one-way mirror while observing the trainee hypnotizing a client in the interview room. Telephone suggestions can be made, and these do not seem particularly disruptive in this setting because the subject is usually occupied elsewhere.

I recommend that trainees get whatever training in hypnosis they can and hope that long-term training in clinical hypnosis is available to them locally. Not only is there value in learning how to use hypnosis in therapy, but the personal skills one develops in the process are even more important and can be applied to all kinds of therapy.

While I emphasize the value of hypnosis in therapy training, I should also identify the negative factors. It seems that whatever is marginal in the field of psychotherapy involves hypnosis—for example: the therapy of multiple personalities and the multiplication of personalities in therapy. More extreme uses also exist: People who claim to have been kidnapped by aliens usually have those memories brought back with hypnosis, and therapists who regress subjects to a previous life to find the cause of a current symptom are hypnotists. In addition, there are people who have false memories about abuse in childhood, and these are usually brought out with hypnosis. It seems obvious that proper training in the techniques and use of hypnosis will help hypnotists avoid the production of delusionary material.

Erickson taught hypnosis not only as a technique for therapy but also as a means of enlarging the imagination. The primary task of a therapy teacher is to succeed in enabling a trainee to be innovative and imaginative in order to deal with the variety of problems encountered in clinical practice. What Erickson taught clinicians through his use of hypnosis was the idea that everything is changeable. For example, a therapist can suggest to a hypnotic subject that a hand will lift by itself. If the hand does not lift, the therapist can suggest that it feels like lifting, or that it is lifting without the subject being aware of it, or that the subject could think of it as lifting when it is not. Or the therapist can suggest that the hand is becoming heavier instead of lifting, and by encouraging this belief he or she is thereby defining resistance as cooperation.

A therapist's attitude toward a symptom can be equally imaginative when he or she has been trained in hypnosis. If, for example, a woman who suffered from headaches without a physical cause came to a therapist trained in hypnosis by Erickson, the therapist would immediately think about how her perception of it could be altered. For example, the therapist could suggest to her that the headaches can stop—or that they can occur intensely for a few seconds rather than for hours—or that she has the headache but doesn't feel it, or that she has amnesia for having it and therefore doesn't anticipate having another one. The therapist could also suggest to the client that she could (1) see the headache on a screen and then view it objectively, understanding its meaning, but not feel it; (2) forget the headache by imagining a frightening tiger instead; (3) go to sleep and have both a dream and a headache that slowly vanish upon awakening; or (4) replace the headache with some other use of her head, such as listening to music. The therapist could also suggest that the client think of the headache as a spectrum of color that can move outside her range of perception (meaning that although the headache exists, it cannot be felt). Or it could be suggested that the client develop another self which experiences the headaches occasionally, so that it is only this self, and not the client, who experiences headaches.

A therapist's suggestion to a client can be a directive to suddenly change a behavior, or it can be a bit-by-bit approach, such as "geometric progression," which Erickson liked to teach. Applying this variation of hypnosis to the woman who suffered from headaches, a therapist trained by Erickson might ask her to have one second without a headache today, two seconds tomorrow, four seconds the next day, and so on; in quite a short time those seconds would become hours, days, weeks, and years. (I can recall Erickson saying that if one wants a fast change in therapy, it is best to begin slowly.) The therapist could also ask the client to describe the headache and could then incorporate into a hypnotic suggestion imagery that is compatible with the client's own description of the symptom. For example, if the client reports that she has tunnel vision when the headache arrives, the therapist can make the tunnel vivid by suggesting that it be transformed into a gold mine.

It is helpful for the therapist to take into consideration the function of a client's symptom. If the therapist of the woman in our example suspects that her headaches serve the purpose of enabling her to avoid some duty, he or she could incorporate that purpose into the hypnotic suggestion—for instance, by teaching the client to merely pretend to have the headache, thus preserving its function but eliminating the pain. The therapist could also incorporate a family therapy approach, for example, by using the husband's or mother-in-law's influence to change the woman's headaches. Somehow, the way Erickson taught would free the imagination—of both clients and trainees.

There was another aspect of Erickson that was important to me: He had a sense of humor that pervaded his approach. Therapy can be a grim business, and a sense of humor helps us survive. On the tapes of our conversations the laughter is sometimes so loud that it causes distortion.

3

THE TRAINEE

When selecting therapy trainees who will be taught how to change people, academic achievement is usually not relevant. Having a B.A., M.A., Ph.D., or M.D. does not in itself qualify a person or reveal any potential as a therapist; it just means he or she sat in classes and passed tests. One may find in a therapy training program social workers, psychologists, nurses, psychiatrists, educational psychologists, school psychologists, marriage and family therapists, guidance counselors, hospital aides, addiction counselors, massage therapists, and acupuncturists. Which profession best prepares a person to become a therapist? There is a curious situation here. Educators in each profession train clinicians in the way they consider best and ignore the ideas and procedures of other professions. Yet if a social worker respects the work of a psychiatrist doing therapy, then he or she is saying that psychiatric training is what should be done, even if social workers do not get that kind of training. If psychiatrists agree that educational psychologists should be licensed as therapists, they are saying their own training is not essential, since educational psychologists have not had that.

It has been demonstrated that trainees with only a high school education can become expert therapists with outcomes equal to those of therapists with graduate degrees. At the Philadelphia Child Guidance Clinic in the early 1970s, Salvador Minuchin and I instituted a program to teach trainees to work with poor families. It was a time when we had to either teach the middle-class therapists what it is like to be poor or teach the poor to be therapists. We did both. The program was for 2 years, and training took place 8 hours a day. The trainees selected had no academic background beyond a high school education, and they knew nothing about psychological problems or therapy. They were taught family therapy, and they worked with both poor and middle-class families. They were given live supervision with every interview. They only knew what we taught them about therapy (at first we kept them separate from the staff so that they would not be influenced by others.) Basically, we were training people in family therapy who had never been trained in individual therapy.

At the end of 6 months these trainees were mixed in with staff members, who had been envious of the trainees' intensive supervision since the staff too was trying to learn family therapy. Staff members' ideas were different and interesting. I recall a meeting where a staff member presented a videotape of a family interview. The staff competed with each other in making comments about the dynamics of the family. The non-professionals listened politely. They did not comment until they were asked for their opinion. Then one of them said, "Wouldn't it be better to ask the family to take their coats off?" It was then that we noticed that the family members were sitting in their chairs huddled in their coats.

An outcome study confirmed that the clients of the nonprofessionals did as well as those who had been in therapy with staff members.

SELECTION CRITERIA

The supervision of therapists with different previous training does not particularly differ on the basis of profession. Far more important is whether a therapist loves and respects people in distress. Nevertheless, a major issue is whether the trainee will be able to be licensed to work as a therapist. To train someone who cannot be licensed is impractical. Quality training is expensive, and the outcome should be worth the investment. Therefore, trainees should be chosen who will make their living doing therapy and who will be able to pass on to others what they have learned.

In the selection of trainees, what is more relevant than profession or academic status is the professional context of the person, for example, whether the trainee is simultaneously involved with some other supervisor or another school of therapy; whether the trainee works in an inpatient unit (which is particularly relevant to the range of therapy techniques he or she will need to learn); and whether the trainee is in personal therapy or has had considerable therapy, particularly with an individual focus (in which case he or she will be difficult to train in a socially oriented approach). Unlearning must be done with most trainees—and must also be done with supervisors who have had extensive personal therapy, have taught in ideologically rigid settings, or work on inpatient units.

When trainees are in a situation where loyalties are divided between their supervisor and their colleagues, there are special problems. For example, the seeming incompetence of a trainee when doing an interview might be explained by the trainee's nature, character, or past. However, it may also be that the trainee is caught between two training authorities and feels that he or she must work one way to satisfy a teacher in academia (or perhaps a personal therapist) and another way to satisfy a training supervisor. The result is paralysis, which may be mistaken for incompetence.

TYPES OF TRAINEES

For practical purposes, trainees can be divided into at least three types: *novices*, *groupers*, and *ideologists*. Trainees of these types can be taught, but some are more difficult than others and require special efforts.

The Novice

Novices are the easiest to train. They are eager to learn and acknowledge that they need training. Often, they have graduated from academic training programs and have been given difficult clients with whom they are expected to work without supervision. Finding that they do not know what to do except to say, "Tell me more about that," or "How do you feel?" they seek out training in how to do therapy.

In a way, the less trainees know, the easier they are to train in a new approach to therapy. (This does not mean they should be dumb. A dumb trainee is one of the most difficult to train.) They do not come with preconceptions that make it difficult for them to accept the therapist's ideas. The reason novices are easiest to teach is not only because their ideas have not yet solidified, but also because they are usually not imbedded in a network of colleagues who may be offended if they take a new approach, It is characteristic of large cities that new therapy ideas are accepted slowly, if at all (while professionals and clients usually think of themselves as being in the avant-garde and leading the field). One explanation is that the networks of trainees, therapists, teachers, and spouses are so tight that any change in ideology or practice would be disruptive to a number of people. Change is best avoided.

However, problems do arise with novices. Sometimes they try to compensate for their inexperience by being arrogant, an attitude that must be corrected, or they can be frightened and surprised that a family in therapy would pay attention to them. Novices discover the power of being in an expert's position and must learn how to use that power. Sometimes young novices try to act older than they are. I remember the first time I saw quite young people in training. It was at the University of Kansas, where James Stachowiak was training graduate students. I watched a young therapist interview a family whose problem daughter was not much younger than the therapist herself. The parents were expected to listen to this young woman who was not married and knew little about families or raising children. I was accustomed to older family therapists, who had personal experience with marriage, some of them having been married several times. Out of the discussion that day came an obvious plan to have the therapist define a position to work from: She needed to say to the parents something like, "You know more about marriage than I do, certainly more about your own marriage, but I have been trained to be an objective observer and can therefore be helpful to you in that way." The parents accepted that position. It also became evident that if a young therapist allows it, older parents will be helpful by improving because they are protective. Obviously, therapists should use whatever they have—youth, old age, experience, or inexperience.

Sometimes novices become so involved in academic views that they forget they are doing therapy. They can become fascinated by theory—especially when they do not know what therapeutic action to take.

Another problem with novices is that they sometimes have difficulty recognizing a serious problem. Some novices have only learned from books and not from observing different kinds of severely disturbed patients. Often they have not had experience in mental hospitals and are therefore unfamiliar with severe problems. If they are taught a therapy technique for a particular problem that minimizes its severity for strategic reasons, novice therapists sometimes underestimate the problem's severity.

Being a novice doesn't necessarily mean that the individual is inexperienced in conducting therapy. The type of novice who is easiest to train is the person who is experienced as a therapist but who concedes that he or she is without experience in the particular therapy approach of this training. For example, a trainee who has skill in gathering information, making clients feel comfortable, managing a private practice, etc., may wish to learn ways of doing brief therapy. He or she doesn't have to be trained in the management of therapy but in how to tell clients what to do to change.

The Grouper

A "grouper" is a trainee whose therapy experience has been with artificial groups in group therapy. These therapists present a special problem and are even more difficult to train than ideologists. Their clients in group therapy have been strangers who meet together under their guidance. The group may be organized around a symptom or being incarcerated together. Such groups typically deal with substance abuse, sex abuse, or domestic violence; often, group membership has been court ordered and so is compulsory.

The problem in training groupers is that they have a way of working that gives them satisfaction even if their clients do not change. Not only are groups lucrative and fashionable, but the group process itself compels involvement. It is also one of the easiest therapies to learn. The therapist need only bring together a group of strangers and ask them how they feel about being there. An occasional "Tell me how you feel about that" will spur the group on, requiring the therapist to know little about what to do to change people. Of course, group therapy advocates would protest this statement and insist that group dynamics are complicated and that the group therapist must be profound and skillful, particularly with confrontations. But if a group therapist sits down with a family, it is apparent that he or she has difficulty doing an interview, doesn't know what to do to produce a change, and is confused about setting a goal. Rather than focus on the organizational problem, groupers focus on the emotional and internal processes of clients. Their skill is in getting people to express what is on their minds—whether this resolves their symptoms or not. They typically have great difficulty seeing an organizational connection between people, and they prefer to focus upon how clients perceive and feel about people. They have difficulty with the idea that their clients may function differently in the group than they do in relation to their family and social situation. It is assumed they need to understand how they see the world and then they will be able to change in the real world.

The organizational hierarchy of a family is difficult for groupers to grasp because they have worked only with groups of people who are unrelated to each other and for whom there is no hierarchy of membership. Groupers are confused about the status positions of family members and are sometimes confrontational and provoking, not realizing that these approaches are inappropriate in a family interview, since family members must go home and live together. In artificial groups there are no adverse consequences to these techniques because group members usually don't share a home. Most group therapists assume that their task is to bring out members' secrets and painful experiences of the present and past. When this is done with families, the consequences are quite different. To train a grouper not to focus on catharsis, secret sharing, and repressed ideas is a difficult supervisory task.

An example of the artificiality of group therapy can be seen in the consequences of the trend that brought business executives together into groups to help them "grow." The typical group therapist did not recognize that there are important differences between executives who work together and those who are strangers from different companies. It was at first not fully appreciated that expressing one's opinions and feelings to a stranger has different consequences from expressing oneself to one's boss.

Supervisors and trainees must make a choice of whether to be purist or eclectic in the therapy approach. In the early days of family therapy there was a question as to whether family therapy was to be used along with other therapy approaches or whether it was a new way of thinking about and doing therapy. If it was based on a different view of human beings, techniques from other therapies would have to be abandoned. Therapists who grasped the new view based their therapy on a unit of two or more people. This meant giving up group therapy and individual therapy, with the focus on the interior of the person. By the 1960s, it was possible to separate out the "purist" family therapists from those who were trying to be fashionable without changing their ideas. A key indicator of whether a therapist had grasped the new systems view was whether he or she still did group therapy. Obviously, group therapy isn't based on the idea that a symptom has a function in a social group; it's a therapy that's concerned with the interior of each individual in the room. The systems and group ideologies are incompatible. (It should be emphasized that the value of self-help groups is not the issue here. There are endless numbers of such groups, and many seem to provide people with satisfaction. The issue here is the training of therapists for family therapy who have a background in group therapy and thus have a special approach and ideology.)

An important contribution of a purist is that he or she forces others to take a position. Purist family therapists thought that a new idea had arrived in the world, one with considerable consequences for what therapy would become. Other family therapists thought that they could mix all the ideas together and avoid taking a position. When purists condemned them for accepting the eclectic mix, confrontation developed. It was a time of change, and out of this confrontation new ideas developed.

Don Jackson, a major family therapist, was a purist in the field of family therapy. Once he realized that family members were systematically locked together and that therapy should deal with that, he changed. He resigned from the American Psychoanalytic Association, he removed the couch from his office, and he began to see whole families together in therapy at a time when hardly anyone was doing that. In the early 1960s, Jackson was invited by the American Group Therapy Association to speak on family therapy. At that time, family therapy was beginning to be popular, and the group therapists wished to consider it a form, even a subtype, of group therapy. In his keynote address Jackson said flatly that group therapy and family therapy have no relation to each other in theory or in practice. Family therapy is focused on the systemic behavior of people who have a history and a future together whereas group therapy focuses on the individual and is based on an ideology that has produced nothing new in the way of theory. The untimely death of Jackson (in his 40s) was a considerable loss to the family therapy field because he was courageous in taking a position on the issues. When I organized a meeting in his honor after his death in 1968 I brought together 46 people from around the nation who considered themselves family therapists, I found among them only a few purists like Jackson.

Because they don't know how to work with people related to each other, groupers often resist interviewing family members together. If a husband is ordered to therapy for beating his wife, the grouper will want the husband in a villain's group and the wife in a victim's group, often recommending that membership in these groups last for years. Groupers consider it wrong to see such marital partners together—even if they are living together and seeing each other all the time. To persuade such therapists to change their orientation to a family orientation can be difficult. Even when they see whole families, groupers do not conceive of the family as an organization.

There is a pessimism in the field of group therapy (perhaps because of the therapeutic results) that makes it difficult for a group therapist to work with an optimistic view. In substance abuse therapy, group therapists tell their clients that they are incurable, that they will always be abusers, and that they can only restrain themselves (and worry that they will relapse). For example, a 23-year-old heroin addict was brought in with her family for therapy: When seen alone, she wept and said she had a disease and was incurable (she had been told so in several drug treatment programs). The family therapist had to work against that idea to get her to accept herself as a normal person with a problem. Groupers often do not realize the effect on a family or in the community of the stigma of a disease label. In another case a father came into therapy with his family and said he was an alcoholic. When asked when he last had a drink, he said it had been 26 years. His family had defined him as a defective person all that time in spite of his being sober the entire lifetime of his children. In some cases, perhaps such a stigma is necessary to persuade a client of the severity of a problem, but when it is applied irresponsibly because of an ideology, it can cause suffering. Rather than call a client's addiction an incurable disease, it is better to say that the therapists have consistently failed in their approach with the client.

It can also be difficult for a grouper to accept the idea that family members should help each other stop taking drugs or drinking. They have the idea that such a person is an "enabler." The argument is that addicted individuals must reach bottom to change and that their families should not interfere with their fall. For example, a man in his 40s who was living with, and being supported by, his mother was asked by a family therapist to bring her into an interview when he mentioned that she was an alcoholic. She not only drank but was ill, and the drinking was going to cause her death. The son refused to have his mother come in. He said that to try to help her would be wrong because that would make him an enabler. He was willing to let her die rather than break the Alcoholics Anonymous rule against helping. The idea that family members should not help each other with substance abuse came from a period when therapists did not know how to organize families to help. With a competent therapist, a family has far more positive influence on an addicted member than does a group of strangers.

Residential Programs

Another factor that makes training of groupers difficult is the fact that they often work in residential programs. Because of the nature of the setting, it is difficult for therapists in such programs to join parents in a family approach to therapy. They become fond of their clients, particularly when they are unhappy children who spend a great deal of time in therapy and see little of their parents. Typically, groupers blame the parents for the client's problems, and when they meet the parents, they are often unsympathetic and critical, thus disempowering the parents. Parents respond to this negativism by withdrawing, and therapists take such a reaction as evidence that they are poor parents. Therapists tend to side with the client they see alone (It is helpful for a supervisor who sees that a trainee dislikes a particular family member to arrange for the therapist to meet alone with that person. This usually improves the situation.)

When parents have had a child removed, it is difficult for staff to join with them to guide the child. Often, too, groupers have had substance abuse problems themselves and are in conflict with their own families. They prefer to rule parents out of the therapy. When groupers change and do outpatient therapy, they discover that they must learn how to motivate clients in ways quite different from the ones they used when they had authority over someone in custody.

Although groupers are difficult to train in a family-oriented therapy, this does not mean that it cannot be done. Many recover.

The Ideologist

Ideologists present special problems during training, although they are easier to train than groupers. Usually, therapists in graduate school become immersed in theories and different ways of classifying what is wrong with people. They learn to make textbook distinctions between schools of therapy. They say things like, "Is that structural therapy and not strategic therapy?" They think if the teacher can formulate a difference, they will know better how to do therapy. When they begin to do therapy, they find that changing people requires a different way of thinking. The action is not in the mind but in the real world. I recall an intellectual therapist being educated one day by a young man who had a way to intimidate his parents—when they disagreed with him, he would sprinkle gasoline around the foundation of the house and then sit on the front steps lighting matches.

Most therapists recover from being ideologists when they face the problems of therapy and become more interested in the skills involved than in the ideas. Some trainees never get past the theory stage, and it is the supervisor's task to help them. An example of this is one pointed out to me years ago by Don Jackson. We were discussing the therapists stuck in object relations theory, and Jackson pointed out that that was a stage for many of them. They studied Fairbairn and worked out a theory of object relations in their head. Once they could do that, they could then transfer that way of thinking from object relations to people relations. Of course, today some supposed family therapists are still trying to salvage object relations theory by calling it a form of family therapy.

Often, ideologists are reluctant to accept the idea that they should change their clients. Their focus is on understanding them (and sometimes sharing that understanding with them). This type of ideologist likes to think of therapy as architecture, not as carpentry. Such therapists want to be profound and prefer the philosophical aspects of therapy (sometimes they resemble French intellectuals). The ideologist is an enthusiast for any new fashion in ideas. When psychoanalysis was the most popular ideology, the ideologist was deep in the psychodynamic theory of repression. As fashions change, these therapists get involved in theories of the aesthetics of therapy or in discussions of epistemology, constructivism, dissociative processes, or cognition. It is difficult for them to focus on concrete problems, such as a child's refusal to go to school or an adolescent's refusal to eat. They like diagnostic categories like "borderline personality disorder" and will dwell on them despite their irrelevance to therapy. It is the ideologist who makes a supervisor realize that therapy was born in the university and can be thought of as an intellectual way of life rather than a set of procedures for bringing about change. The goal of ideologists is to have intensive seminars rather than focus on changing unhappy people. They carry to an extreme the natural enthusiasm of educated people for theoretical understanding and new discoveries.

The novice, the grouper, and the ideologist are, of course, not the only types who come for training. They are just the easiest to recognize. There is also the "compulsory trainee," who is in the training program because his or her educational institution requires it. Often such trainees don't want this training or don't want to interview in a one-way mirror room in front of colleagues. They sometimes raise ethical reservations about the use of one-way mirrors in therapy—when, in fact, their motivation for doing so is a fear of exposing their poor interview skills to others. Their attitude is not a helpful one. It is difficult to persuade such trainees that they will do best in the training process if they think of themselves as novices with a lot to learn in this new approach. Whether or not they ultimately use the family therapy approach, the most contemporary therapy (it's only 30 years old), they should have a grasp of it.

THE ACADEMIC INFLUENCE

The Training of Social Workers

There are special issues involved in training members of the different helping professions, each has its advantages and difficulties.

Social workers are conducting most of the family therapy in the United States today and therefore are represented most often in training programs and therapy workshops. A merit in training them is their knowledge of social systems and their awareness of the practical needs of clients. They are taught how to obtain resources when families need them, and they have experience with poor families as well as middle-class ones. At the turn of the century they earned a reputation for knowing how to deal with families; clinicians of other disciplines who wished to learn about family therapy would seek out a social worker. However, clinical social workers were not learning about family therapy in their own training: Instead, they were learning individual therapy and wishing they could be psychoanalysts (the largest group in psychoanalytic treatment were social workers for quite a period of time since having that therapy gave them prestige in their profession). Family therapy developed outside the social work field, but in the last decade the enthusiasm of social workers for family therapy has increased and is reflected in the curriculum of programs for the training of social workers.

The problem in social work academic training has been that there is more emphasis on the history of social work than on how to change a client in therapy. The curriculum tends to be unsophisticated and narrow. The clinical training social workers receive is in their placements rather than in their academic work. Fortunately, social work schools are changing, and quite a number teach therapy and even train students in family therapy in one-way mirror rooms. This is in part because of pressure from social workers who discover after graduation that they don't know what they need to know about how to do therapy and must seek out postgraduate private training. Ideas in the universities about supervision change more slowly than do therapy practices in the field. Psychodynamic theory is still being taught in social work schools.

Let me cite an example of how social workers were trained in the past. A few years ago a young social worker consulted me about the case of a small child who not only set fires but did so wherever he went. He would toss lighted matches into the wastebaskets in the child psychiatry clinic. The social worker told me that she was just out of social work school and had no training in what to do in therapy, particularly with a fire setter. When she admitted this to her superiors, they told her not to worry because the child would be tested and at a staff meeting she would be instructed what to do. Actually, in that child psychiatry clinic, as in many other child clinics, the same approach was always taken: Someone saw the child in play therapy while the social worker saw the parents. Indeed, this child was tested, and both his parents were interviewed. Several weeks—and several fires—later, the staff met to consider the case. The testing of the child was reviewed, as was the interview material gathered from the parents. It was concluded that the child should be diagnosed as a fire setter, and there was a discussion of the psychodynamic meaning of fire setting. At the end of the case conference the director of the clinic, who was conducting the staff meeting, stood up and said, "Well, it's obviously an oedipal problem." Everyone left the room. The social worker sat there and began to cry because she had learned nothing in social work school to help her with this problem and she had learned nothing from the staff of the child psychiatry clinic.

Fortunately, there was a happy ending to this story: A psychologist, a behavior therapist, passed the empty conference room and saw the social worker crying. He asked her what was wrong, and when he learned what had happened, he said that something ought to be done about the fire setting. "Let's see. To set fires, the boy must light matches," he reasoned, thinking like a behavior therapist. He suggested that the social worker have the parents give the boy a penny for every 10 unburned matches he brought to them. The social worker was pleased to have some definite plan of action, and she proposed this to the parents. The parents were pleased that finally someone was giving them something to do to solve the problem. The boy liked the idea and brought quite a number of unburned matches to his parents. He stopped lighting fires while the therapist dealt with family issues. What a contrast that intervention was with what was taught in social work school. Yet times

are changing, and social work supervisors are now trying to find training
in how to teach contemporary family therapy so that they can learn what
to tell trainees to do to solve clients' problems.

The training of marriage and family therapists is still new enough to
have an uncertain academic curriculum. In the best schools, students are
taught how to conduct therapy to manage a variety of child and family
problems. In the worst, students are trained only to pass the state
licensing examinations and therefore learn only that material and not
how to practice therapy. The designers of the curriculum do not seem to
see this new profession as an opportunity to drop the irrelevant issues
carried over from therapy training programs of the past. Instead, they put
great emphasis on conversation supervision and require many hundreds
of hours of that. If trainees get live supervision at all, it is in their
placements.

The Training of Psychologists

Psychologists are primarily trained in research methods; until recently,
their clinical training was secondary and lacking in prestige. However,
clinical training is now being taken quite seriously partly because it has
become lucrative as a profession—there are even efforts by psychologists
to limit the number of clinical psychologists in the field by increasing the
difficulty of licensing examinations. Academic training in psychology
lasts for years, but not much of that time seems to be spent learning
therapy techniques. There is extensive study of abnormal psychology but
no instruction on how to bring about change in those abnormalities.
Psychologists attend lectures about and study all the different therapy
schools and their histories. The result is often a therapist with an eclectic
point of view who assumes that he or she should not take a personal
position about how to do therapy because that would be too narrow.

The merit of a background in academic psychology is that the
training is intellectually broad and can induce a scientific attitude. After
such training, graduates are able to examine ideas in the field of therapy
critically. If they have an internship in a mental hospital, they can see and
get personally involved in the care of people with severe problems, an
experience that will help them recognize such problems when they appear in private practice.

Psychologists can develop a handicap as therapists if the research
attitude they learn permeates their therapy approach. Researchers learn
to be objective and neutral; not personally involved with the experiment,
and they are devoted to not influencing the data. Exactly the opposite is
true in therapy. A therapist needs to be personally involved, not neutral,

and the main therapeutic task is to influence the data and change them. Shifting from one position to the other can be difficult for many trainees with a background in psychology. If they are given training in behavior therapy, they learn to be more active. Often, they try to retain the influence of their academic training by conducting therapy based on cognition. They feel that it is compatible with their academic learning to use therapy to enforce rationality on their clients.

Of course, there is variety among university psychology departments in this country and no orthodoxy. The ideology of one department can differ quite remarkably from the ideology of another. Therefore, a clinical supervisor should make no assumptions about how a trainee psychologist will be. For example, years ago I lectured at New York University, and the discussion with the students was entirely within a psychodynamic framework. Later the same day I went out to Stony Brook to give a seminar, and I heard no psychodynamic ideas mentioned at all; the discussion there centered around a disagreement between Skinnerians and Wolpeans about the best approach to therapy. Yet only a few miles separated the two universities.

The Training of Psychiatrists

Anyone who has taught seminars in therapy to psychiatric residents over the years has seen a steady deterioration in therapeutic focus. (For a discussion of issues involved in training psychiatrists to do therapy, see Chapter 7.)

CONCLUSION

Often, when students ask me what type of profession to enter to learn to do effective therapy, I have to point out to them that it depends on the particular school and department they will be associated with. Having seen so much disappointment, I usually advise them not to expect to learn much about doing therapy from their academic training, to think of the degree as a union card that allows them to practice as a therapist, and to expect disappointments in the relevancy of their academic work to their clinical training. For several years it has been necessary after acquiring an academic education for therapists to go for private training in institutes unaffiliated with universities. Perhaps times are changing, but one must keep in mind that universities are organized to save the best of the past, not to change their curriculum with every passing whim.

There is another aspect of trainees that is becoming more of an issue.

Supervisors are expected to train therapists from different socioeconomic classes and ethnic groups. Therapy training is no longer a middle-class monopoly. The poor have entered the field as clients and also as trainees, and a variety of national origins is represented among those who come for training. When teaching in the United States, many Europeans and Latin Americans attend training programs. Recently there has been an increase of trainees from all over Asia. It is fortunate that clients of different ethnic groups can increasingly turn to therapists who share their cultural background and who therefore can better understand them. The interest of minority group members in conducting and seeking therapy is also a benefit to supervisors, who can gain greater understanding of the culture of minority clients and can apply this understanding in their own clinical practice.

A primary concern with trainees from other countries is the issue of language. Sometimes trainees speak little English and must become observers at the same time they are learning the language. Or a foreign-born therapist may have learned to speak excellent English outside the United States but may lack an understanding of idioms and slang. Most foreign-born therapists are somewhere in between.

A structural, organizational approach to family therapy makes it possible to resolve problems when there is minimum communication between therapist and client. If one wishes to do therapy that requires a discussion of the meaning of life, the communication is of course, more complex. I recall the training experience of an Italian psychiatrist who hardly spoke English and who treated an African American woman who spoke a dialect that was difficult for him to understand. The supervisor encouraged client and therapist to struggle amiably to understand each other. Live supervision made it possible to offer suggestions to clarify misunderstandings. In the process, the child problem was resolved, and the two adults came to enjoy each other. The mother's problem with the child was partly the fact that she and her own mother could not agree. The therapist helped the two women resolve their differences since he understood aspects of their problem from his experience with similar conflicts between his own mother and grandmother in Italy. When the focus is on the family, there are cross-cultural similarities that make treatment possible by a therapist whose culture differs from the client's. The particular behaviors for dealing with a family of a different culture might be new to a therapist (such as which member should be asked what the problem is), but the family structure and system will be familiar.

Often, having a member of an ethnic group behind the mirror as a trainee will help all the trainees recognize the cultural differences when they observe a family. For example, a therapist in the room with a Latin American family was discussing the husband's macho behavior as something he learned from his father and grandfather. This individual view was corrected by a Hispanic therapist behind the mirror who pointed out that many Latin American women like their husbands to be macho because they are more predictable and can be manipulated more easily. Such behavior is therefore encouraged by some women. This view assumes a current social function for the behavior, not a past cause.

Having experience with a family in poverty, or any ethnic group, often helps a therapist to better understand middle-class families, and supervisors should therefore expose trainees to poor clients. For example, sometimes a therapist will hear the following comment from a mother in poverty who interferes with her husband when he is dealing with their adolescent son: "I'm afraid my husband will kill that boy." The therapist, after hearing this, can more easily understand the true feelings of a middle-class mother who says, "I'm afraid my husband might express hostility toward our son." What she means is that she's afraid he will kill him. Working with the poor in the 1960s helped many supervisors orient themselves to new ethnic groups and widened their views of therapy. (See Chapter 4 for further discussion of cultural and economical factors in treating clients.)

4

THE CLIENT

Therapists today are expected to deal with all types of problems and clients. It is the supervisor who prepares them for that impossible task. In an ideal program, trainees would be given experience with every type of problem, family, and life stage, either as therapist or as an observer behind the one-way mirror. In reality, of course, the selection of clients for trainees to treat or observe is limited but an effort should be made to present clients who differ in age, socioeconomic class, and ethnicity. Exposure of trainees to as great a range of psychopathology as possible should be achieved. It is hoped that after training, therapists will be expert in certain areas and will have a working knowledge of others so that they will be able to deal competently with the multitude of different problems their clients will bring. A therapist is not fully trained if he or she must refer out to someone else a client with a particular problem. Trainees do not learn properly if they anticipate routinely passing difficult cases on to someone else.

If the goal of therapy training is to teach therapist how to solve the problems of a broad range of clients, supervisors must emphasize that referrals are not usually made to other therapists. However, there are times when referrals to other professionals with particular technical skills are necessary, such as, for example, when a client has a learning disability, needs to be detoxified, or requires a medical examination. A referral is also appropriate if the client simply can't get along with the therapist and wants another one. There should not be referrals for special types of psychological problems, such as childhood problems, sexual difficulties of a couple, severe drug addiction, or psychosis. Trainees should learn that they must deal with whatever problem a client presents. Clients improve best when they realize that their therapist is determined to solve their problem and will not give up easily. Though they may feel trepidation, trainees should expect to struggle in one hour with, say, the problem of a runaway adolescent and in the next with an abuse problem in an immigrant family in which only one member speaks English. Trainees might be uneasy about fielding every type of problem, but in the long run they will realize the benefits of this training approach. The variety of problems their clients will bring to them over the course of their career is so great that the more experience they get during training, the better off they will be.

WHO SHOULD HAVE THERAPY?

There are two views of therapy: One is that therapy is for a person with a problem, a handicapped person who cannot solve a difficulty. The other view is that therapy is good for everyone, since those who have it are helped to develop and become a better person than they would otherwise be. Each supervisor and therapist must choose which view to accept. This decision has consequences.

If one thinks therapy is for people who cannot solve their problems themselves, one does not take everyone into therapy. In a first interview one might advise the client that therapy is not needed. On the other hand, if one thinks of therapy as designed for self-enrichment and consciousness raising, one takes everyone into therapy because everyone can improve. Of the many consequences resulting from the point of view adopted, there are two primary ones: hierarchy and stigma.

Hierarchy

If one thinks more therapy is better, more therapists are involved in treating the members of a family and the hierarchy that results among therapist and family members then becomes an issue. If every family has as many therapists as possible for as long as possible, confusion rather than change can result: The parents are in marital therapy while each child is in individual therapy and the family is in family therapy.

From the other point of view of organizational, not individual, development, the more therapists the worse the outcome. A covey of therapists are likely to be pulling the family apart by relating in different ways to each family member. Conflict among the therapists is inevitable since there are legitimate differences in view. The family members each use their own therapist to support them against the other family members. Meanwhile, each therapist is often following an ideology that assumes that the goal of therapy is to help the individual family member to a higher level of being, and the influence of each therapist on the organizational and hierarchical problems in the family is underestimated. In an extreme case the individual therapists can pull parents apart to the point of divorce, confine adolescents in psychiatric institutions or juvenile halls, and place children in foster homes—in short, they can dismember the family.

When there are several therapists involved with a family, it can be helpful if they have an executive session to see if they can at least reach consensus on the goals for the family. For therapists to do this requires reasonable sophistication. This problem is changing with the introduction of managed care, since a number of therapists will not be financed.

Stigma

Stigma results from the view that therapy is only for the emotionally handicapped. In this view, those in therapy have something wrong with them that they cannot solve on their own. Indeed, since the general public still thinks that only defective people go to therapists, being in therapy can have consequences at work or school or if one runs for public office. Moreover, there seems to be less stigma attached to those who are in family therapy or couple therapy than to those who are in individual psychotherapy.

Even the length of therapy is affected by whether one thinks therapy is good for everyone or necessary only for certain people. If therapy is a form of self-development, the more of it the better; that is, long-term therapy is better than short-term therapy. But to those who hold the opposite view, a person in therapy for years is considered more defective than one who received brief therapy.

Each therapist must choose which general view of therapy is best. If a therapist chooses the view that more therapy is better, his or her clients should be advised not to try to run for president.

SOCIOECONOMIC DIVERSITY

A young man in a family interview said, "Just before Pig went to jail, the Dude came by and sold me some smoke. I found that comfortable and better than drinkin', but I ain't got no Jones." The therapist conducting the interview understood the young man's discourse perfectly. Many therapists—and their supervisors—would not.

When dealing with people of different social classes, a therapist must be flexible. Sometimes the problem is learning to understand a dialect different from one's own. Sometimes one needs to learn the expressions of members of a different class or generation. If the therapist doesn't understand a client family's dialect, the family will usually shift into the therapist's language (and will sometimes go back to their more natural dialect when the therapist leaves the room.) Therapists should not pretend to understand clients whose dialect is unfamiliar to them, which is patronizing, but should convey the fact that they are doing their best to comprehend what is being said.

Dealing with the poor means understanding not only the language but the culture of poverty as well. I once supervised a young man in his early 30s who had been raised in poverty and was doing therapy with poor families. A 50-year-old mother who had brought her child for therapy asked his advice about other matters in her life. The woman had been going with an 80-year-old man for several years. He gave her money when she needed it and once paid for a trip to a funeral that was important to her. Perhaps because of her therapy, she had recently begun to enjoy life more. For example, she started going out with a man in his 50s, and they had fun together. The woman asked the therapist whether she should stay with the 80-year-old man or take up with the younger one. I assumed the therapist would advise her to go with the young man and enjoy life. However, the therapist came out of the culture of poverty and thought differently. He advised the woman to stay with the 80-year-old. This man had proved himself to be reliable and helpful (he had paid the way to a funeral) whereas the reliability of the 50-year-old, whom the woman had known only a short time, was unknown. This is an example of a supervisor learning from a therapist-in-training what it is like to be poor.

It can be difficult for a middle-class therapist or supervisor to grasp what it is like to live in poverty. It wasn't until the 1960s that psychotherapists began to treat the poor, and serious adjustments in the traditional therapy approach had to be made to deal with this population. One change was that therapy began to be less intellectual and more behavioral, a change that helped many intellectual therapists enter the real world.

The poor tend to be out of fashion today, compared with the 1960s, but we will have them with us always. It is equally important that trainee therapists learn to deal with middle- and upper-class families. While the family system and structure from one socioeconomic class to another may be similar, the therapy relationship and interventions are different. It is the supervisor's task to understand class structure well enough to be able to guide the therapist whose client's social class differs from his or her own.

Fortunately, clients who are rejected by clinics because they do not have money or insurance are always available for training programs. It is essential that the therapy these clients receive be of the same quality as that extended to those who enjoy greater economic security. There should not be second-class therapy for clients who are seen by therapists-in-training.

WHAT OF ETHNICITY AND NATIONALITY?

When a high school in Maryland recently had a multicultural festival, 180 different ethnic groups were represented. Although a therapist's practice might not include clients from that many different cultures, at least half that many might end up in his or her office. It is the supervisor's task to prepare therapists for this diversity. When psychotherapy was born in the 19th century, consideration of such cultural diversity in the client population was not part of the training program. In fact, resistance to a multicultural view existed. I recall attending a meeting of the Psychoanalytic Society of San Francisco in the 1950s to hear a lecture by an East Indian psychiatrist. Starting with the premise that psychological problems are different in different cultures, he described a subculture in India where parents could only quarrel about their eldest son; that is, if they had any differences of opinion about anything, these had to be defined as a disagreement about the son. The psychiatrist pointed out that a therapist had to take such a cultural rule into account when considering a patient's Oedipus complex and that the oedipal conflict of a patient in this culture would necessarily be different from that of a patient in Vienna. When the psychiatrist finished, the head of the psychoanalytic society stood up and said that he thought the speaker simply did not understand the oedipal conflict and should therefore not be speaking about it and imposing his views on others. Many analysts in the audience were as embarrassed as I at this rudeness to a thoughtful colleague. Perhaps this sort of attitude is why psychoanalysis died.

Therapy is no longer a monopoly of the mainstream culture. Both clients and therapists are culturally diverse. I have supervised therapists from Scandinavia, Germany, Argentina, Puerto Rico, Israel, Italy, and Japan, to name a few, as well as Americans of different ethnic backgrounds.

Sometimes a family from a particular culture can be provided with a therapist from the same culture. When such an arrangement is possible, there is greater understanding in the interview. Of course, a client and therapist might be of the same ethnic group but of a different class or religion, and these differences can cause difficulty. For example, a man who seemed to be out of his mind was recently brought to an emergency room. He was speaking a language none of the staff could understand. They finally concluded that he was Cambodian and hired a translator to find out what was upsetting him. The translator proved to be a Vietnamese who hated Cambodians and refused to speak to the patient. Such problems are no longer rare.

Training Therapists to Treat Clients from Other Cultures

The supervisor's task is to train therapists to do therapy with people of different ethnic groups and to be flexible enough to shift gears from one therapy session to the next. For example, in one therapy hour a therapist may conduct an interview with a young American couple who think of themselves as equals, and in the next hour the therapist might see a Middle Eastern husband who refuses to be interviewed with his wife. Supervisors must help trainees learn to do therapy in spite of limitations in their knowledge of a client's culture. There are two possible positions to take: the anthropological or the family systems approach.

The Anthropological Approach

Supervisors can model themselves on anthropologists and learn all they can about the culture of the clients seen by their trainees. They would then be able to alert trainees to cultural differences. For example, in one case a therapist defined as typical a problem of a depressed adolescent brought in by his mother. The mother mentioned almost in passing that her son was suffering because she had been witched. The supervisor then had the therapist shift focus to talk about who was witching her and for what purposes. It was finally hypothesized that the woman was attempting to reunite with her family in the country she came from. She believed that the only person who could save her from being witched, and her son from his depression, was a shaman back home. That is, the unhappy mother wished to be reunited with her family, and the need for a shaman to treat her son's depression was making the trip home necessary. As always, the family will educate the therapist who listens.

Gregory Bateson taught psychiatric residents (many of whom had never read a book that wasn't a medical book) by offering them a wider view of the world. I recall one day that he was lecturing on a culture whose members believed that they did not make laws but only discovered those that were already made by a higher power. One of the residents said indignantly, "Those people are crazy! Of course people make laws!" Bateson was gentle with him, not even reminding him that in his religion it was assumed that God makes laws.

Therapists must have enough anthropological knowledge to appreciate cultural similarities and differences, but the therapist's task is still therapy, not academic understanding. For example, one might be dealing with a case where a young couple marries and moves into the home of the husband's parents. The wife comes under the domination of her mother-in-law, and there is conflict. An American couple in such a situation might be encouraged to move out of the parents' home. In a culture where this arrangement has been the norm for a thousand years, such a solution wouldn't be considered proper, and some other solution would need to be found. Therapists must adapt to certain basic premises of a culture. If a husband will not sit down with his wife and treat her as an equal, the couple can be seen separately and their problems worked out. The goal is not to make members of the client family behave like members of the ethnic group of the therapist but to respect the clients' culture and still resolve their problem.

The therapist who takes an anthropological view would study kinship systems, childhood toilet training, eating habits, attitudes toward elders, and so on. The problem is that therapists simply don't have time to research the ethnic group of each client they meet. Even if they do, they can't learn the culture well enough to be acquainted with all its nuances. Even anthropologists limit themselves to one or two cultures—and can spend a lifetime studying those. A reflective therapist can spend many hours with a family learning their views on the meaning of life, but the goal of therapy is to bring about the changes clients seek, not to teach the therapist about their culture.

The Family Systems Approach

The other alternative in teaching trainees how to handle cultural diversity is to generalize from a family organizational view and to use one's knowledge of family systems to find ways to intervene helpfully with individual families. Primarily, one assumes that it is often the presence of cross-cultural difficulties that brings an immigrant family into therapy. For example, a typical problem in such a family is that the members have different reactions to their migration to the United States. The children learn English quickly and want to follow American customs whereas the parents want to preserve their cultures, including its traditions on child rearing. Often, the wife can find work but the husband cannot. Her work and her association with American women makes the wife more independent than she was before. The husband may feel that his patriarchal rights are threatened and he beats up on his wife. When the police intervene, the husband learns that in America it is against the law to beat one's wife. The judge recognizes the situation, and refers the family to therapy. What does the therapist need to know about a family's culture to solve such problems? They are not unique to a particular culture. The client family could be from India, with the father wearing the turban of a Sikh; a village in Guatemala; or a town in Portugal. It's the adaptation of the family to a new culture that's the essential problem.

Therapists should know as much as possible about the particular culture of a client family, but they can't know all cultures and must simplify. It would be nice if trainees and their supervisors were authorities on the culture of every client, but this is not likely. The task is not to be an authority on a family's culture but to understand the family well enough for therapeutic interventions to be made. Supervisors should know how to help trainees conduct an interview courteously with clients of different cultures and should teach them to have a respectful attitude toward all the ways people live and think in the world. Since the therapist cannot know every culture, he or she must explore the client in therapy. It is appropriate to say, "I don't know the ways you think about these issues. How would the problem be dealt with if you were back in the country where you were raised?"

However, some families, particularly Asian families, might not comment if the therapist makes a social blunder because they wish to help him or her save face. When one asks the family how this problem would be dealt with in their country of origin, a discussion can often lead to a plan that takes their usual ways into account. This inquiry also allows the client to politely correct the therapist's understanding of the situation by implicitly comparing it with their own approach.

What is important is the relationship of therapist and client. In some cultures those who seek help want an authority to tell them what to do; they do not want an exploratory discussion. In contrast, members of another culture would oppose an authoritarian therapist and seek a milder form of consultation. In some Latin American cultures the father has such power that the therapist can lose a case by ignoring him, and in some cultures it is improper to discuss adult issues when children are present.

A family systems approach to psychological problems makes it possible to resolve problems when there is a minimum communication between therapist and family. One needs to recognize that in many cultures the father is in authority (or the family treats him as if he were); when that authority breaks down because of cross-cultural influences, the family has a dilemma, which can take various forms. And in every culture there are conflicts with adolescents and with people marrying outside their caste or class. There are also parents who are divided over how children should be disciplined and siblings who are struggling with each other.

Although the psychological issues involved in a case may seem simple, resolving them may not be. In one case an Italian mother brought in her 15-year-old daughter, with whom she was having a conflict over dating. The daughter wanted to begin to date, and the mother felt she was still too young. The daughter, tall, blonde, and attractive, insisted that every 15-year-old girl she knew was dating. The mother decided that she needed family support in this matter and had taken the girl to Italy, at some expense, to have her mother, who had always been very strict with her, speak to her granddaughter. The grandmother said she thought it was wonderful that girls were dating and having fun at 15. The angry mother returned to America and was now seeking the help of a therapist to solve the problem.

Supervisors who teach therapists to approach each family as unique are less dismayed by ethnic diversity than those who use the anthropological approach. If one designs a therapy for a particular family, class and cultural differences become less important and solutions grow out of the exploration of the family's problems.

A therapy approach that focuses on family problems and assumes that psychological symptoms arise from conflicts in family structures is most successful and requires less knowledge of the premises of a culture. Supervisors with this approach must teach their trainees to recognize typical family problems and to follow the courtesy behaviors necessary to join with clients from different ethnic groups. Therapists must also be taught the skill of making tentative interventions and observing the client's response. Anxious trainees would prefer to have rigid rules and standard procedures to follow, but supervisors must teach them an experimental attitude. Each family, regardless of its culture, is different, and therapists must experiment to determine how to join a particular family, how to understand its problems, and how to offer ways to resolve difficulties.

Often a therapist and client deal with their communication difficulties with good humor and enjoy the therapy. Sometimes that collaboration is lost with a translator inasmuch as the family tends to orient toward the translator rather than the therapist. (Generally, it is not a good idea to have one family member translate for the others. It is better to provide your own translator.) Sometimes the translator screens ideas from the therapist. It can also be a problem if the translator is not skilled in being neutral. When different languages are involved (including sign language with a deaf client), the supervisor must encourage patience from everyone concerned. If basic respect for everyone is built into the training program, trainees from different cultures will respect each other and will respect the ways of their clients.

Case Example

An example of a difficult case that came out well illustrates the range of possibilities with ethnic therapy. A young Japanese therapist who spoke little English and was shy about speaking it attended a training program. We arranged for her to sit with other trainees behind the one-way mirror while her English improved. (She was expected to ultimately do therapy with families in English). She observed and was able to follow the cases.

One day a Japanese family who spoke little English was referred. The Japanese trainee was pleased to see them and to do therapy in her own language. She provided a translator for the supervisor and trainees behind the mirror.

It was learned during the first interview that the young couple had one child and that therapy had been ordered by the court because the husband, an extremely successful businessman, had beaten his wife. The husband was angry at the court-ordered therapy and puzzled as to why it was against the law for a man to hit his wife. He was also especially sensitive since he felt humiliated by having been arrested. The therapist had the problem of being an expert in charge of this couple's therapy while also being a woman in a culture where women tend to be considered secondary.

The therapist managed quite skillfully to join the husband in his difficulties, winning his respect for her as a therapist, and to encourage the wife to not allow herself to be beaten. The anger of both spouses subsided with the therapist's interventions. Meanwhile, behind the mirror the supervisor struggled, with the aid of the translator, to understand what was happening. The translator became interested in the dialogue and often forgot to translate.

Fortunately, the therapist needed little guidance, having learned a great deal from the interviews she had observed. This case involved brief therapy, and in the follow-up it was found to have been successful in that violence did not occur again in the household and the couple got along more amiably. The therapist impressed her supervisor by the way she ended the therapy: In the last session she introduced a ceremony during which she brought out a small bottle of champagne with which she and the couple toasted each other in a pleasant farewell. Perhaps a therapist who wasn't Japanese would also have had a successful outcome with this case, but it wouldn't have been conducted with such grace and style. This case is an example of how being immersed in the culture allows a therapist to avoid resistance and gain acceptance for his or her interventions.

THE CLIENT'S AGE

Trainees naturally prefer to do therapy with people they feel comfortable with. This usually means clients of a certain age group or those with a particular type of problem. A surprising number of therapists say they sought therapy training because they wished to help adolescents. However, young therapists are sometimes at a stage in life where they have difficulty with parents, and that bias may intrude in their work. Often they recover from such a bias when they have children themselves. I recall one child psychologist who said that after he adopted two infants, he wished he could apologize to the mothers he had advised in the past, that is, when he had no real idea what problems there were in raising children.

Trainees should have firsthand experience treating children, adolescents, adults, and the elderly, as well as the whole range of diagnoses. No longer can one confine therapy skills to a single age group. Since children hardly live independent of others, a child therapist should also be able to deal with the child's depressed father or with a difficult family network. The parents of troubled children often have difficulties themselves, and the therapist needs to know how to provide them with help.

Treating Children

Working with children requires a special ability to communicate. It helps to have a few of one's own. Sometimes a child is the presenting problem, and he or she sometimes is just brought in as part of the family. In either case the therapist must be able to join the child, and the supervisor must offer guidance in how to achieve that. I recall hearing a therapist once say to a 5-year-old, "Have you considered the derivation of your problems?" That therapist had never met anyone under 21, and one of the tasks of his training was to introduce him to children.

One of the purposes of teaching trainees about play therapy is to help them communicate with children in an imaginative way. Play therapy might not change a child who has a problem, but it educates the inexperienced therapist. (I recall Nathan Ackerman, a family therapist and child psychiatrist, telling me that he didn't think play therapy ever changed a child. When I asked him why he never said that publicly, he replied that it would just hurt the feelings of a lot of his colleagues who didn't know what else to do with children.)

A child with a symptom may be expressing the issues in a social network and deserves to be interviewed in that context. However, the therapist must also respect the needs of the particular child and must help the child out of his or her difficult situation. When I was trying to impose the ideas of family therapy on him, Milton Erickson said, "Sometimes a child builds a stack of blocks to please his parents, and sometimes he builds a stack just to please himself."

There are ways for a supervisor to help a therapist join a child. Seeing the child alone and sitting on the floor with him or her can be a good beginning. Having the child do something is important. It is helpful to have a blackboard in the therapy room so children can express themselves with it and thus give the therapist information about their abilities and limitations. Therapists who were previously schoolteachers often have superior ability to organize a group of siblings so that progress can be made with the parents.

Most child problems are somewhere between two extremes: The child is withdrawn and must be coaxed out, or he or she is agitated, even violent, and must be restrained safely. Most children's problems express the conflicts between the adults who must deal with them. For every pair of adults in conflict about a child (e.g., mother and father, father and grandmother, mother and schoolteacher) there is increased disturbance and hyperactivity in that child. Generally, supervisors help therapists learn how to join children by being playful about it. Watching other therapists with experience with children is especially helpful.

Trainees must learn not to neglect the social situation in which the child's problem has a function, yet they must not allow this focus on the social situation to leave the child's personal problems neglected or unsolved. A training program must teach therapists to deal with children of different ages in their social contexts. This does not necessarily mean bringing the social context into the therapy room immediately, as in an interview with the whole family. Therapists must learn different ways to enter a family. If an adolescent is misbehaving in an attempt to bring the parents together, it might be wise to avoid immediately addressing that issue. For example, one depressed adolescent was unwilling in a family session to say what was on her mind. It was apparent that her parents were in conflict about her and in distress themselves. The supervisor had to decide how to approach this problem. When the daughter was seen alone, she revealed to the therapist that she had had sexual relations with her boyfriend and that he had broken up with her immediately afterward. She was upset about this, but her major concern proved to be uncertainty about how to deal with the boy when she saw him again. That issue was addressed in the therapy first, and family issues were dealt with later. Whatever the structural problem in the family, a child or adolescent can have quite personal immediate concerns that must be dealt with. For example, an adolescent girl who is having problems as a way of bringing her parents together is still suffering and needs help herself before she can help them. The supervisor must teach the trainee how to decide priorities.

Treating the Elderly

The art of supervision is to help therapists learn to change a situation while focusing on the particular needs of the person with a problem. Bringing in the individual alone and later bringing in the family can be appropriate with many age groups. An 84-year-old woman was expelled from her retirement home for misbehavior. On a visit to her son and his family, she sat down on the kitchen floor and refused to leave. She was referred to therapy by a crisis center. Although a therapist for such a case might ordinarily wish to bring in the people relevant in the elderly woman's life, including her son and his wife and children, it seemed evident from the referral source that the son and his wife were furious with the woman and that she was angry at them. The elderly woman referred to her son's wife as "the worst daughter-in-law that ever lived." To bring them all together initially did not seem wise. When the woman was seen alone, it was apparent that she wished to live with her son and his wife, rather than live alone. By getting herself expelled from the retirement home and refusing to leave her son's home, the woman was trying to force her son to take her in. However, the son and his wife did not want her to live with them. They already had the wife's 90-year-old parents in their home, a fact that also made the elderly woman angry. If they could take the wife's parents in, she wondered, why couldn't they take her in? It was evident that the family was at the stage of life where something had to be done with an elderly parent, which is one of the most difficult stages for families to deal with and for therapists to help them with. In this case the therapist managed to help the woman pull herself together and behave in a more reasonable way with her son and his wife. The son and daughter-in-law were then able to enter therapy in a positive way instead of in anger. The family's ultimate arrangement was for the elderly woman to live in a retirement apartment and visit the family for Sunday dinner and participate in the grandchildren's activities. Often in crisis situations it is better for the therapist to have clients take one step at a time rather than have a session in which clients confront each other in anger.

THE CLIENT'S PSYCHOPATHOLOGY

If therapists are to deal in their practice with the whole range of psychological problems, they must have access to as varied a client population as possible during training. It's not practical for therapists to specialize too narrowly. Nevertheless, in reality the clients one sees in a training program, such as in a child guidance clinic, might be radically different from those one treats as the years go by. One might, for example, decide to be only a marital therapist. Yet what does one do if one of the spouses has a compulsion or is depressed? The spouses might also be in conflict over a problem child, and mothers-in-law have been known to be central in some marital problems. In other words, one soon learns that to try to specialize in one type of psychopathology it is necessary to pretend that other people are not involved. It's better to have a broader view of therapy and to learn a greater variety of skills. A trainee might be more expert with certain problems but should still be able to deal with the wide range that appears in therapy.

It can be a problem when colleagues specialize in one type of therapy, for example, group therapy or therapy that prescribes medication for every problem. Supervisors must train therapists to deal with these colleagues in such a way that a client's care is not sacrificed to disagreements between professionals. For example, a therapist has several choices when a psychiatrist begins to prescribe medication for an individual when the therapist is working with the person or the family. One choice is to go along with the medication, even if it causes problems. For example, a mother whom the therapist is trying to empower can be defined as defective if she is medicated, which makes it difficult for her to take charge. Often, this choice is labeled the psychoeducational approach. For example, a psychiatrist medicates someone defined as schizophrenic and relies on the social worker to persuade the family that the person is incurable and must always be on medication. The social worker in this way allows the psychiatrist more time to see more patients, but the main purpose of this arrangement is that it allows cooperation between psychiatrist and the social worker or another therapist. In contrast, when social workers take the sensible position that people defined as schizophrenic are curable with therapy without medication, they come into irreconcilable conflict with psychiatrists and the medical establishment. Since there is not evidence that schizophrenia is physiologically caused (no one has received the Nobel prize for discovering a physiological cause of schizophrenia), the client is being sacrificed to harmony between colleagues. Not only do antipsychotic drugs not cure people, but they prevent normal behavior and cause neurological damage, such as tardive dyskinesia, in a large number of cases. Social workers and psychologists who participate in this arrangement are as responsible for the damage as the psychiatrist who medicates. Perhaps the worst part of this crime is that authorities insist that persons defined as schizophrenic and their family must believe the problem is incurable and will never change, a belief that blocks these persons off from all therapy. There is little evidence that these pronouncements are true and ignored evidence that they are not.

If a therapist doesn't want to accept the incurable view and doesn't want to be in a conflict with a psychiatric colleague over basic issues in such a case, the logical thing to do is to abandon the client to the psychiatrist. However, this view makes difficulty for the supervisor of a training program. Trainees should learn how to do successful therapy with the most difficult cases, which involve psychotics, drug addicts, and retarded persons. One learns more by treating a family of a severely disturbed person than one does from any other type of family. To accept the premise that such people are incurable and must be drugged or put away is simply not acceptable. Supervisors are often left with the possibility of treating only two types of such cases: those clients for whom medication was prescribed—unsuccessfully—over the years, and those for whom medication was stopped because the resulting brain damage is evident and embarrassing to the medical establishment.

Of course, supervisors should provide not only difficult cases for trainees but also easy ones. A case or a type of intervention should be chosen on the basis of the needs of a particular trainee as well as the needs of the client family.

THERAPY IN THE HOME

An increasingly common setting for doing therapy is the home. This has many merits but can be a problem where supervision is concerned. Live observation is awkward, but one can record a session and review it later. Another alternative is for the therapist to go to the client's home with the supervisor and introduce him or her as a colleague who might or might not get involved in the discussion. Then the supervisor can sit out of the way. This arrangement allows the trainee to conduct therapy with a supervisor available to protect the family from therapist errors.

Therapy in the home provides the therapist with more information than in the office. Office visits bring out public behavior, and one can be quite surprised to discover how different people are at home. It is helpful to take a tour of the house with the family, noting the sleeping arrangements and whether the family uses the dining room or eats in front of the television set. (Sitting down together in the office for an hour or more is a unique experience for some families. Since such families rarely sit down together to discuss something, particularly a problem, they must be advised how to do so.) Since the home atmosphere is so informal, with members free to move about or go to the bathroom if they become uncomfortable during the therapy session, the therapist must provide some kind of structure. The first step is usually to say, "Do you mind if I turn off the TV while we talk?" When trainees deal with a severely disturbed family, I have always asked them to get invited to dinner in the home. This occasion is not to conduct therapy but to interact with family members in a social situation. The therapist learns a great deal from such a visit, and the family relates to him or her more intimately because the therapist has extended himself or herself. One of the first families I treated was composed of two parents and a daughter who had been diagnosed as schizophrenic. I saw the family a number of times in my office, and then in a crisis I visited their home. I discovered for the first time that the mother was a compulsive housekeeper whereas the daughter kept her room an absolute mess. During my visit I saw the daughter drop a cigarette on the floor and rub it out with her foot. Mother looked away in despair. I would never have gained that information in the office. If one thinks like an anthropologist, seeing a family only in the office is like asking a primitive tribe to come on a cruise ship to be studied.

WHAT IF PEOPLE HAVE TO GO TO THERAPY?

A contemporary issue in therapy is the large percentage of cases that involve compulsory therapy, that is, therapy ordered by the court. These cases often involve abuse (including substance abuse, physical abuse, and sex abuse) or other illegal acts. Because judges have now discovered therapy and often sentence people to that experience, supervisors must teach trainees how to deal with clients who do not wish to come for therapy but do so to avoid something worse. (This type of therapy will be discussed in detail in Chapter 11.)

SUMMARY

It is evident that therapy training is becoming more complex. The supervisor must teach the trainee how to deal with families of different classes, ethnic groups, and stages of family life, as well as with the whole variety of symptoms of psychopathology. A family whose culture differs from that of their therapist educates the therapist about their culture while the therapist attempts to bring about a change within a setting where help and change have quite different meanings from those in the family's own culture.

If families would remain in recognizable form, the task of therapy would be easier. However, it seems that the focus on the family began in the 1950s just as families began to disintegrate in divorce. Half of marriages break up, and many second marriages end in divorce as well. Families are becoming increasingly complicated. Children must adapt to parents, and then to separated parents, and then to a new parent, and often to yet another one. Meanwhile, the number of grandparents is multiplying also, and these individuals have unclear rights and responsibilities in regard to the children. If one hypothesizes that the problems of children occur when adults are in conflict about them, the opportunities for such problems multiply with the increase in multiple marriages and their breakups. Sometimes it is helpful to ask a child in therapy to go to the chalkboard and list the people in his or her life, marking who is related to whom and who is in charge. The confusion becomes evident.

With this increasingly complicated family situation a therapist is forced to think of each family constellation as unique; certainly, one cannot follow a therapy method constructed for an ideal family. Supervisors must teach therapists how to focus on and develop a plan for each complex family constellation. In this constantly changing social situation, supervision becomes more complex (and more interesting). Trainees have the opportunity to adopt an attitude of benevolent curiosity about how different people live.

5

WHAT TO LEARN,
WHAT TO TEACH

A supervisor conducting a training program on therapy must take a position on a variety of issues: whom to teach, what to teach, how to teach, and how to make sure it is taught. There are broad issues and quite specific ones that all supervisors must address for themselves; there is no orthodox supervision that we can simply adopt.

SHOULD ONE TEACH EVERYONE'S
THERAPY OR ONLY ONE'S OWN?

During their training, therapists must decide whether they will learn a variety of therapy approaches or concentrate on only one of them. Will they read and observe many different approaches or choose one and specialize in it? Their supervisors have an even more consequential decision, since many therapists will be affected. Should a supervisor teach different schools of therapy or only his or her own? If a supervisor teaches all therapy approaches and presents them as being of equal value, the trainees will become eclectic, which would be unfortunate. To be eclectic means never taking a position or having a firm opinion on anything. Yet if a supervisor teaches only his or her own approach, then the trainees may remain unaware of other ways to do therapy, some of which are quite popular, and they will be thought of as ignorant.

As in the teaching of other arts, one way to deal with this dilemma is to teach a particular approach well and then later teach other approaches, selecting out what is valuable. It is recommended here that the supervisor begin by teaching his or her particular approach. When the trainee is grounded in that approach, other methods and ideas can be taught. It is impractical, but students should undergo the personal experience of doing therapy before they read textbooks. Once they are able to work well in a particular approach, they have something to fall back on when they are faced with an unusual case. Trainees need security. Milton Erickson argued that each subject hypnotized is unique and needs a unique approach. However, when I was a beginner, he advised me to memorize a hypnotic induction. Then he told me not to use it but to adapt my approach to each subject. The memorized induction is there to fall back on if one becomes nervous or is uncertain what to do. An anxious therapist typically goes back to what he or she first learned in therapy training. This is sometimes a pain to later teachers who have a different approach.

It is also wise to help students avoid becoming stereotyped in their thinking. Orthodoxy is as bad as eclecticism. Once one teaches, for example, the idea that a symptom has a social function and trainees have learned ways to change the social situation, one should describe a therapy based on quite a different principle. This will loosen up the thinking of the students. For example, when students become rigid in their thinking about family therapy, I like to introduce a videotape of the treatment of a client who had a lifelong bee phobia and was cured in 16 minutes (with a year-long follow-up) by Steve Andreas with no emphasis whatsoever on the function of the symptom.

DOES ANYONE STILL WANT A METHOD?

A supervisor must decide whether to teach a method of therapy or train therapists to devise different therapy procedures for each case. Trainees prefer a method because that's easiest to learn; whatever problem the client presents, they can do with this case what they did with the last one. Teaching a method is the simplest approach and requires the least from the teacher. Everything done is a standard procedure; the supervisor doesn't have to be innovative. The main objection to a method is that only clients who fit it can benefit from therapy. With so many kinds of clients and problems being seen today, it seems obvious that therapy must be designed for each client. What if one chooses a particular symptom and claims there must always be a special method for that? For example, one might insist that for an adolescent who threatens suicide, a therapist could always follow a "threat-of-suicide method." Yet suppose one adolescent is threatening suicide because the parents are breaking up, another so she can stay in a foster home and not go back to her family, and a third because she has just been rejected by her boyfriend. How can one method apply to all situations?

It's true that following a method is convenient for a therapist. It's not surprising that therapists search for methods and argue that they have the best one. Sometimes they take one minor aspect of a traditional idea and say they have found the true method of therapy. For example, they may claim that emphasizing solutions or emphasizing the positive or having a conversation is a new method. While following a method makes therapy easier for a therapist, it is least appropriate for a client with a problem.

I recall in the early 1960s being told by a training psychoanalyst that he was disappointed with the new crop of young psychoanalysts. He said that when he became an analyst he was part of a rebellion against traditional psychiatry. At that time analytic ideas were revolutionary. With the success of the psychoanalytic movement that changed. The young analysts entering the field in the early 1960s were no longer rebels with new ideas; they were seeking orthodoxy and respectability. They wanted to be taught what to think and what to say and what color suit to wear. They weren't interested in new ideas but on behaving correctly. The emphasis on a method was killing the movement.

In my own experience, when psychoanalysts gave up the couch and became family therapists, they often kept all the worst ideas, including (1) that one should follow a method in family therapy, (2) that training should consist of personal therapy, and (3) that families are really inside the client's head and a matter of perception.

Let me give an example of the power of the method approach: In 1959 I gave a lecture with Don Jackson at a meeting of the American Academy of Psychoanalysis, which was an organization of psychoanalysts who were trying to save that pastime by introducing new ideas. The academy wanted a presentation on family therapy, which was barely a few years old at that time. The analysts were shocked to hear for the first time about interviewing whole families (they would not even speak on the telephone to a patient's relative). The use of the one-way mirror also upset them since it revealed confidential interviews to other therapists.

A few months later I was invited to Philadelphia, where a group of psychoanalytically oriented therapists who had been at that meeting were starting to do family therapy. They invited me to watch from behind the mirror. The client family consisted of a mother, father, and 18-year-old daughter. The father had had sexual relations with the daughter, who was then put in a psychiatric hospital (which was typically done with incest victims in those years). The interview I observed was conducted just before the daughter was to go home for the weekend for the first time since the hospitalization. Everyone seemed to be worried about what might happen at home, but no one could bring up the topic of incest. The interview was rather bland; the two cotherapists in the room were not accustomed to initiating a topic.

After the interview the therapists said they wished that the family had brought up the incest problem since it seemed to be on everyone's mind. I said that I thought the therapists should have brought the issue up and that the girl might need protection. They replied that a therapist only responds to what clients say and doesn't initiate subjects. I said that if they had to follow that rule, they should at least help the family bring it up and that the therapist could, for example, go behind the mirror after asking the family members to talk together about their concerns. (Families often talk about important issues if the therapist leaves the room. In fact, sometimes they avoid talking about a subject because they are waiting for the therapist to leave the room.) The therapists objected to my suggestion but not for the reasons I expected. They told me that family therapy didn't include leaving the room during a therapy session. I replied that it was possible for the family therapist to be either in or out of the room. I pointed out that one of the original family therapists, Charles Fulweiler, had a well-developed procedure of letting the family talk together while he watched from behind the one-way mirror, and entered the therapy room at times, and that others had tried it and found it helpful. The staff informed me that what I advised wasn't family therapy.

This group had only been doing family therapy for 3 months, yet already they had a method and an orthodoxy: A therapist only interviewed the whole family, no individual sessions were allowed, cotherapy was always done, therapists never initiated a subject but just responded to client's comments, and a therapist never left the room to observe from behind the mirror. They had managed to attempt something entirely new, yet they felt obligated to take on all the dead weight of a method. They seemed to me to be concerned both about being fashionable and about avoiding antagonizing the powerful psychoanalysts in their community. Yet in trying to pacify them they took the least valuable contribution of the psychoanalytic tradition. Of course, they claimed that their family therapy, which they called "intensive family therapy," was deeper than any others, which they characterized as shallow. They also attacked me for being "manipulative" because I recommended planning what to do in therapy.

How persistent this "method" approach can be is illustrated by the way one member of this group, a decade later, invited me to watch a therapy session with a new approach. From behind the one-way mirror I observed a group of married couples and cotherapists. This was not a new approach to me since a number of group therapists had been seeing families or couples in groups. As the therapy session unfolded, it seemed to me to be a desultory conversation concerning complaints about children. After the session I asked the therapist who had invited me, a prominent family therapist, why they were seeing couples in groups like this. I added that it seemed to me that interviewing each pair of spouses separately was more effective and that others had reached that conclusion. He replied, "This is what we're doing now." I asked why they were doing it. Had they found they had better outcomes by seeing couples in groups? As if puzzled by my question, the therapist repeated, "But that's what we're doing now." I then asked if cotherapists were more effective than one therapist, adding that no one else seemed to have found that to be the case. "But cotherapy is what we're doing," he explained.

These therapists considered the primary defense for what they were doing to be the fact that they were correctly following the method—not whether or not they should be using one. I thought my questions were relevant, but they did not. It is better for a supervisor not to be a methodist.

WHAT THEORIES SHOULD BE TAUGHT?

Just as therapy practice should not be stereotyped, so neither should theory be allowed to become an orthodoxy that limits the range of therapy interventions. From the many theories the supervisor must select the most helpful ones to teach trainees. (It is hoped that supervisors are able to teach theory in such a convincing way that it is obvious that their own approach is the correct one.) Even before the supervisor decides which theory is best, there is the issue of the kinds of theories to consider. There are at least three different types of theories the supervisor must clarify and take position on: (1) a theory of normal behavior, (2) a theory of why people do what they do, and (3) a theory of change.

How About a Theory of Normal Behavior?

In the 1960s I was conducting a research project in which I used a variety of tests and experiments for families. I was trying to answer the following questions: Are families with members with symptoms of different kinds different from each other and different from "normal" families? Is a family with a delinquent son different from a family with a normal son? Is the family containing a person who is diagnosed as schizophrenic different as an organization from other families? If psychopathology is a product of the family, then families with a problem member should be different from "normal" families. An investigation of this question required selecting normal families for a control group, but how does one determine whether a family is normal? I began by asking clinicians to examine a sample of families and select the normal ones. They found none. They were only able to find abnormality. That's what they were trained to find. Because they had no criteria for it, they could not find normality. I ended up testing about 200 families that had been randomly chosen from a high school. If no family member had been arrested or had been in therapy, the family was defined as normal. Actually, I defined normality for a family as the ability to handle its own problems and not call on the community to deal with them. (Once when I had a family experiment I wished to try out on a family. I called a friend whose family seemed average and explained that I needed a normal family to try out an experiment. When I asked if they would come in, they agreed. However, a few hours later the wife telephoned and said they would not come in. She said they weren't a normal family because their daughter was about to go to college and everyone was upset and quarreling. I then realized that "normal" could only describe a family that was not at the moment at a crisis point in their stage of family life.)

Today clinicians still have no criteria for normality. One cannot say, "I will treat this abnormal person or family and make them normal," because no one can agree on normality. In a curious way normality is being defined as not being described in the American Psychiatric Association's *Diagnostic and Statistical Manual of Mental Disorders*, the DSM-IV. Everything not in that bible is normal.

What Good Is the DSM-IV?

As the clinical field becomes medicalized and bureaucratized the DSM-IV is increasingly used by institutions, insurance companies, and researchers. For therapists this is a misfortune. The categories used and the implicit ways of thinking about human beings in the manual will handicap any therapist. If therapists must categorize individuals, they should choose categories that guide them to a therapeutic approach. Not only does the DSM-IV not offer such guidance, but by its very nature it expresses hopelessness about change.

Diagnosis is important because those who classify have power. A classificatory scheme builds an ideological system and thus controls how people think about the topics classified. I am reminded of a case that Joseph Wolpe presented to a seminar of therapists. He described a woman, her anxieties, and his treatment. After a period of time during the discussion of the case a psychiatrist spoke up after hearing the woman's name mentioned. He said that he himself had treated the woman for several years, but that he had not recognized her from Wolpe's description of her. Thus, the language one therapist uses can make his or her clients unrecognizable to other therapists.

It seems taken for granted today that therapy is more successful if the therapist has a positive view of the client. They collaborate better together, and the client feels there is hope. The DSM-IV describes people in such a negative way that no clinician would want to have as a friend anyone categorized in that manual. The people described there aren't nice. Who wants a pal who is "borderline"?

Supervisors should teach the DSM-IV only for practical reasons, that is, because people are forced to use it and because one must learn the language of one's colleagues. It can also be taught by using it to illustrate how not to stigmatize people.

Given the variety of classes, cultures, ages, and problems represented by clients, it would be better not to strive for a category of normal. What is normal is what each individual or family organization considers acceptable. When a person does enter therapy, it might be because his or her stress and problems are greater than those of others or it could simply be that the therapist a person was referred to was more available and persuasive than the therapist someone with similar problems was referred to.

A Theory of Why People Do What They Do?

The bulk of clinical literature is not about how to change people. It's about how to diagnose them and how to explain why they are the way they are.

We should all begin by accepting the fact that a theory of motivation held by clinicians is not the same as a theory to explain people in other settings. Why people on the street behave as they do is one issue; why clients in therapy behave the way they do is quite another. Theories appropriate for a therapist who is setting out to change someone are not theories about how normal people live and do what they do. Therapy theories and theories of how to live are quite different, just as theorizing about how to raise a normal child is not the same as theorizing about how to cure a problem child. These theories should not be confused.

As an example, I recall a psychiatrist friend who had a party in his home for his colleagues. His 8-year-old son wandered into the living room drinking milk from a baby bottle. The father couldn't get angry with his son's inappropriate and childish behavior, exposed in public, because he was following a theory that one should not in any way repress a child. He had taken the unfortunate theory of repression, which was designed for people in therapy, to mean that his own child should be allowed to express everything, no matter how infantile. We now have a generation of children who were influenced by therapists who confused the therapy context and the context of ordinary living.

This brings up the question of what is the best theory for thinking about people in therapy? Let us accept the fact that the therapy situation, which is a context designed to change people, is different from other social situations and that theories that apply there might not apply elsewhere.

Involuntary Behavior

What is the typical client behavior that clinicians are attempting to describe? Clients usually do something, or fail to do something, and say they cannot help themselves. They define their behavior as involuntary. Of all the miseries that come to therapy, the involuntary presentation is the most common. Usually there is some extreme behavior that clients say they cannot help. Some people can never bathe whereas others can't stop washing themselves. Some people won't eat and even starve themselves whereas others stuff themselves to obesity. Some are passive and inert, others violent and aggressive. Some are depressed and quiescent, others hyperactive. Some cannot enjoy sex, others can't enjoy anything else. Some married couples can never express anything to each other, and others can't stop expressing themselves. For every individual or family problem there's an opposite extreme. (Of course, not all clients are characterized by behavior they can't help. For example, clients in compulsory therapy often say they do what they do voluntarily and wish to continue. See Chapter 11 for a more detailed discussion of such clients.)

Why would a person do something and say he or she can't help doing it? Why is a person unable to do what other people do and yet not know why? Those with a phobia, for example, say that something just comes over them and that they can't help avoiding certain situations. A therapist must choose a theory that helps explain this behavior and that also recognizes the possibility of changing it. Explanations that make change more difficult should be avoided.

In the 1880s this question of involuntary behavior, as described by Henri Ellenberger,[1] was investigated at length, and explanations were sought. Three main views were offered, all of them having their origins in hypnosis.

The Unconscious. The unconscious was discovered, or created, in the 1880s. It became the explanation of involuntary behavior, and it was

[1]Ellenberger, H. F. (1970). *The discovery of the unconscious.* New York: Basic Books.

explored with hypnosis. It was said that people had unconscious impulses that caused them to do what they did. Since those impulses were unconscious, the conscious mind could only be puzzled over what the person was doing and thinking.

This explanation of problem behavior gained popularity when Sigmund Freud, with the power of his ideas and organizational skills, created a movement based on the idea that the unconscious causes the misery of symptomatic behavior. A theory of change was also introduced. It was suggested that if people became conscious of their unconscious motivations, they would get over their involuntary behavior. A variation on this theme was the idea that feelings can be repressed, or removed from awareness, in the unconscious. It was hypothesized that expressing feelings would make involuntary behavior and ideas go away. People could get in touch with those feelings that had been unconscious if the therapist regularly asked, "How do you feel?"

Should supervisors teach the unconscious explanation of involuntary behavior today? Should they also teach the idea that change takes place if there is awareness of unconscious ideas and feelings? It is a sign of the persistence of this theory that supervisors don't need an example to understand it. Their teachers instructed them in this theory, and their teachers before them were so instructed, and so on.

It would appear that the concept of the unconscious divided at about the turn of the century. A number of practitioners didn't like the idea of the unconscious as a place of repressed ideas. They suggested that the unconscious is a positive force that can offer solutions for people in difficulty. It was argued that if one allows the unconscious to function, a positive end would be reached. An example is the centipede, which walks best if it's unconscious of how it does it. Milton Erickson represented the hypnotists who believed in the positive unconscious. He would say that if he misplaced something, he would not hunt for it, for his unconscious would reveal it to him when he needed it.

The differences in view of the unconscious created quite different approaches to therapy. For example, supervisors with a positive view of the unconscious might tell trainees that if they have an impulse in a therapy session about how to proceed, they should follow it. Supervisors who view the unconscious as a place full of unfortunate ideas would object to such a suggestion; they would say that therapists who follow their impulses in conducting therapy could bring about misfortune because their unconscious has unsavory ideas carried over from the past.

Spirit Possession. A second theory to explain involuntary behavior is the idea that people can be possessed by spirits. A spirit takes over the body and makes people do things outside their awareness and, therefore, beyond their control. This is the most popular worldwide explanation of involuntary behavior; it appears in cultures on every continent. A theory of change was introduced with the idea that the possessing spirit could help the possessor become a healer of others (just as those who had been analyzed often became psychoanalysts).[2] Thus, the negative force became a positive advantage. Hypnosis or trance dancing is often used as a part of the therapy approach. The problem in teaching this view in the United States today is that one would be considered outside the mainstream of therapy—perhaps too far out. (Oddly enough, previous life therapy seems more acceptable to many people.)

Teaching trainees different approaches, if only as metaphors, is helpful. They learn tolerance of others and new therapy techniques. I like to describe to students the work of a Puerto Rican faith healer living in New York. A man once brought his unfaithful wife to him and said he did not want to kill her. He asked the faith healer if anything could be done. The faith healer carefully examined the wife and concluded that she, herself, had not had the affair but that the spirit of a previous wife was responsible for it. (This is not unlike saying it was another personality or an unconscious impulse based on a childhood experience, like sexual abuse.) However, the Puerto Rican healer also offered a solution, not just a theory. He had the couple travel to a certain town in New England, a long way by bus. They were to walk one mile outside that town to a certain tree, in front of which they were to perform a ceremony he had taught them. This ceremony was to exorcise the spirit of the previous wife. Then the couple had to make the long expedition back to the city. Performing the prescribed behaviors was obviously a penance therapy for both spouses, and it rid the couple of their problem.

Multiple Personality. In the 1880s another explanation of involuntary behavior existed: the idea that a person could be possessed by different personalities. In this view, the primary personality has amnesia when a second personality takes over and so is puzzled about what has happened. In other words, the other personalities are outside the awareness of the primary personality. Hypnosis was the main procedure used to bring the other personalities out. This was a popular theory in the 1880s, but it fell out of favor and was largely ignored (except by Milton Erickson) until 1980. Like an anniversary phenomenon, in that decade several thousand multiple personalities appeared; these were recorded and treated. The concept of multiple personality seems too limited to explain the variety of symptoms therapists see in their practice, but some therapists claim their practice is totally made up of multiple personalities.

---

[2]Richeport, M. (1992). The interface between multiple personality, spirit mediumship, and hypnosis. *American Journal of Clinical Hypnosis, 34*(3), 168–177.

Conditioning Theory

Pavlov (who was also a hypnotist) proposed that one could condition animal behavior by offering reinforcements on a schedule. The proper reinforcements could even cause physiological effects. At some point someone, perhaps B. F. Skinner, had the extraordinary idea of applying this conditioning procedure to human beings. It was also realized that the action of the therapist could be the positive reinforcement. This idea gave teachers in clinical psychology something to teach, and generations of laboratory rats and undergraduates were conditioned. Learning theory became a theory of why people do what they do. Involuntary behavior became defined as a product of conditioning, and it was recognized that conditioning can occur outside a person's awareness.

A variation on this theory was developed by Joseph Wolpe, whose technique should be taught to trainees because it is useful for certain purposes. Wolpe experimented with cats. If a cat is frightened in a particular situation, it becomes frightened each time it finds itself in that situation. However, if the cat is exposed to a little bit at a time, it overcomes its fright. Wolpe contributed the idea that a human being could imagine a frightening situation and with a gradual exposure to it could therefore overcome the fright. Wolpe argued that a therapist should avoid making the client anxious, yet he is considered to belong to the same school of thought—learning theory—as those therapists who "flooded" the client with whatever caused the anxiety (e.g., if a client feared bugs, he was to imagine them crawling all over him). Thus, learning theory became broad enough to absorb quite contradictory ideas.

The conditioning approach helped encourage specificity in defining a problem and designing an intervention and taught therapists to be directive. Nevertheless, conditioning ideas had their limitations for therapy.

There is so little orthodoxy today that it is difficult to believe how controversial the behaviorist approach was when it was first proposed. Let me give an example: In the 1950s I was on Gregory Bateson's research project on communication. We were housed in a research building on the grounds of the Veterans Hospital in Menlo Park, California. In the same building were two young psychologists who were experimenting with behavior therapy. There was a weekly presentation of the research going on, and the hospital staff would attend these meetings. The staff—psychoanalysts and the director of training, an elderly analyst—did their duty by coming to the research meetings. One day the psychologists said they wished to present a new idea they were experimenting with.

The two young men talked about learning theory with animals and informed us that the ideas were being applied to patients. They claimed that if therapists wished to have patients behave in a certain way, they should positively reinforce them when they behaved in the desirable way and avoid responding to them when they behaved in some other way. They explained that if a therapist wished, for example, to have a patient express emotions more, he or she should nod and smile when the patient says something emotional and remain unresponsive when the patient doesn't express emotion. They claimed that if a therapist did this for an hour, he or she would have a very emotional patient.

When the young psychologists finished their presentation, the elderly director of training expressed indignation. He said that this was the behavior of a cad. To influence a patient deliberately was wrong, and doing it outside the patient's awareness was absolutely wrong, even unethical. One of the young men defended himself by saying that therapists do this anyhow; they respond positively to a patient who does what they like, and they fail to respond when the patient behaves otherwise. The elderly analyst replied, "If you do it and you don't know you're doing it, that's all right!"

The issue of deliberately influencing clients is still an important one in the field. Should a therapist attempt to do this, and should it be done outside awareness? Or should all a therapist's interventions be revealed? Or is it all right if therapists only influence clients when they don't know they're doing it?

It should be noted that the field of therapy is tolerant to contradictions. Beginning in the 1950s, with the end of psychodynamic orthodoxy, therapists could work in opposite ways without chaos being created. Not only were a number of therapists then working with a family orientation, but psychodynamicists and behaviorists were avoiding collaboration. Psychodynamicists used interpretation as a primary tool, with the goal being awareness of unconscious motivation, at the same time that behaviorists practiced psychotherapy without making interpretations and without even assuming the existence of an unconscious. The psychodynamicists would absolutely oppose giving directives to their clients, and the behaviorists would direct people to change their reinforcement situations. Two therapists working in adjoining rooms in the same agency with patients with the same problem could be taking opposite therapy approaches. The psychodynamicist's goal was not to change problem behavior; if asked about such a goal, a psychodynamicist would say, "No, my job is to help people understand themselves. If they change, that's up to them." To psychodynamicists, eliminating a client's symptoms was unimportant; what mattered was an understanding of the dynamic issue behind the symptom. Behaviorists, on the other hand, assumed that their job was to change people; they considered their interventions a failure if they did not solve a client's symptom. Nor was the client's social context relevant for psychodynamicists; they would not even talk to a client's relative on the telephone. Behaviorists, on the other hand, would talk to mothers and even coach them to change their reinforcements with a child.

What was shared, to some extent, by all therapists, was the psychodynamic idea that the past caused the present problems. The behaviorist thought that past learning led people to behave as they do. The learning theory basis of therapy became more complicated as practitioners moved toward a position of assuming that a client's symptoms are currently reinforced and that those reinforcements need to be changed. Behaviorists also accepted the idea that clients need to be educated by their therapist, although what they taught their clients was different from what the analysts taught theirs.

Faced with these complications, supervisors today must think through the premises they teach or risk ending up with a confusion of contradictory ideas.

Systems Theory

Not all therapy theories come from the 19th century. Some were introduced in the middle of this century. A new theory of the origin of symptoms is the idea that a family is a self-corrective system, the behavior of its members maintaining the system. If, for example, a husband goes too far, the wife reacts. If the wife goes too far, the husband reacts. If they both go too far, the child reacts. That is, any move toward change in the system activates governors to prevent change. Of course, the theory is a bit more complex, but essentially it states that symptomatic behavior is a response to some element in the family system and that the system must be changed if the symptom is to be changed. Those who say that they can't help doing what they're doing are responding helplessly to the actions of other people. Symptoms, then, are part of a repeating sequence of behaviors which the therapist must attempt to change.

This systems idea was introduced at the cybernetic conferences at the end of the 1940s, and from these meetings the ideas spread rapidly into a variety of scientific fields. In psychiatry, the ideas were introduced to a great extent by Gregory Bateson, who participated in the cybernetic conferences put on by the Macy Foundation and later described psychiatric problems from that systems view. (Milton Erickson attended the first Macy conference.) Don Jackson, who became a consultant on the Bateson project, observed that relatives reacted negatively when patients improved, and he proposed the idea of the family as a homeostatic system.[3]

A primary consequence of systems theory was the abandonment of the idea that the past causes psychopathology. Before systems theory a symptom was thought to be caused by childhood experiences and was conceptualized as an interiorized response to the past. A phobia, for example, was viewed as a response to trauma that was somehow interiorized. The systems view argues that the present situation is the critical one in causing psychopathology and that symptoms are appropriate behavior in the current social context. Since the symptomatic behavior is adaptive and correct for the situation, changing such behavior requires that the social setting be changed. With this idea family therapy was born.

The idea that therapy should focus on the present and not the past is still a controversial issue today. Supervisors must take a position on whether symptoms are adaptive. If a client who was sexually abused as a child has sexual difficulties with her husband, is this because she was abused as a child or does she have a relationship problem with her husband? Therapy will be quite different depending on whether the therapist believes the symptom's origin lies in the past or in the present. Another example is alcoholism: Is it caused by a dysfunctional family-of-origin or hereditary predisposition, or does heavy drinking have a cause in the current social situation? A supervisor must have a clear position and work in a consistent way among the inconsistent ideas trainees are exposed to.

The Family Life Cycle

Another concept that developed in this century is the family life cycle. I must take some credit for that. I developed this framework during the 5 years I was writing *Uncommon Therapy*,[4] published in 1973. I was trying to think of a way to present the therapy of Milton Erickson when I realized that implicit in his work is an assumption that there are stages of family life and that symptoms, as well as the goals of therapy, can be placed within that framework.

If a person or a family reaches a stage in the life cycle and cannot get past it, the goal of therapy is to help the client reach the next stage of development. For example, if a woman has a baby and becomes so

[3]Jackson, D. D. (1959). Family interaction, family homeostasis and some implications for conjoint family therapy. In J. Masserman (Ed.), *Individual and familial dynamics*. New York: Grune & Stratton.

[4]Haley, J. (1973). *Uncommon therapy*. New York: Norton.

depressed that she cannot take care of it, how is the goal of therapy for her to be defined? The goal can be to help her understand why having a baby is upsetting to her. Or the goal can be based on the idea that she is at one of the stages of family life and cannot proceed to the next stage, that of successfully caring for her child. Helping her reach that stage becomes the goal of therapy.

It seems apparent that symptoms and psychological problems do not occur randomly in the life of a family; they occur at stages, which can become crises. The stages of the family life cycle are based on the following events: the wedding and the early years of marriage, the birth of children, the beginning of the children's schooling, the adolescence of offspring, the departure of the young adults from home, and old age. The question of why people behave as they do can be partially answered by knowing the current stage of their family's life cycle and viewing it from the perspective of the family orientation that appeared in the middle of the century.

A supervisor is faced with many choices of theory, some of which are the result of inertia in the field. That is, therapists have tried to be fashionable without changing their theories. For example, they may practice "object relations family therapy" but continue to theorize in the same way they always have, believing that problems and their causes are all in the person's head. Therapists also conduct Gestalt family therapy, solution-oriented family therapy, and dysfunctional family therapy, and so on. These family therapies appear in textbooks as if they were new theories of psychotherapy when they are actually simply a repetition of the past. Of interest to academics who must devise classificatory schemes for textbooks, these "new" family therapies have no relevance for practitioners.

Most therapists today accept the idea that the social situation, particularly the family, is an important determinant of behavior. Accepting that fact leads to therapy interventions that are new and successful. Rather than think of "schools" of family therapy, it is useful to imagine a continuum. At one end is traditional therapy, which is based on the hypothesis that the cause of psychological problems is the repressed ideas and impulses in the unconscious and the solution is insight and conscious awareness. At the other end is a purist family-oriented therapy, which is based on the hypothesis that the cause of problems is in the current social situation, which means that the minimum unit toward which therapy is directed is a dyad. Changing the social situation requires action and directives on the part of the therapist. Thus, certain ideas must be abandoned if a therapist is to take advantage of the revolution in ideas introduced by a family orientation.

So far we have discussed the following concepts therapists may choose as the theoretical basis for their clinical approach:

Unconscious
Spirit possession
Multiple personality
Conditioning theory
Systems theory
Family life cycle

There is another theoretical approach, and that is the one this book is about. It borrows some of these concepts and adds others. To understand this approach, we must first discuss the issues a therapist must address when choosing a theory of therapy. Before revealing the theory presented in this book, a test is in order to help readers determine where they are on the continuum from traditional therapy to a sensible family-oriented therapy.

Test

1. Should one do group therapy with artificial groups as well as the family group?
   Yes __ No __

2. Should one explore the client's past dysfunctional family to learn the origins of the problem?
   Yes __ No __

3. Would it matter whether members of the client's family-of-origin, or the person responsible for the client's trauma, is deceased or still alive?
   Yes __ No __

4. Should the therapist initiate what is to be talked about and what is to happen?
   Yes __ No __

5. Should the therapist plan what is to happen in an interview before seeing the client?
   Yes __ No __

6. Should the therapist see the whole family in the first interview whenever possible?
   Yes __ No __

7. Should a client who has had long-term therapy be considered more improved than one who has had short-term therapy?
   Yes __ No __

8. Is the goal of therapy to help clients grow and raise their level of self-awareness?
   Yes __ No __

9. Is it best to assume that problems are based on clients' constructions of reality and their view of their family rather than on what is actually happening in the family?
   Yes __ No __

10. Should the young adult with a problem be placed in a prestigious establishment if the family can afford it (e.g., the Menninger Clinic, Chestnut Lodge, or Austin Riggs)?
    Yes __ No __

11. Should a proper detox take at least 30 days?
    Yes __ No __

12. Is medication valuable because it helps the client communicate in therapy?
    Yes __ No __

13. Should the therapist assume all family members must be treated as equal in their right to comment during a therapy session?
    Yes __ No __

14. Should one think of the world as made up of villains and victims in order to orient oneself in a positive therapeutic posture?
    Yes __ No __

15. Should therapists save clients from colleagues who are tenaciously holding them and using the wrong approach?
    Yes __ No __

16. Can you explain Zen?
    Yes __ No __

On a scale of 1 to 100, being caught up in the errors of the past yields a score of 1 and having a sensible view yields a score of 100. Trainee therapists recovering from their academic education cannot be expected to achieve a perfect score, or even approach it. Any supervisor who cannot answer these questions correctly should read the remainder of this book with care and even review again what is said up to this point. (Those supervisors who achieve a perfect score should write their own book.)

6

THE BEST THEORY

Once we believed that we had to know the truth about what caused symptoms, and what function they served, in order to create a theory to change them. We believed that the real cause of a symptom and the real mechanism of change needed to be found. After a hundred years of the search for truth, years that yielded conflicting conclusions from multiple theories of therapy and intensive, long-term exploration of cases, it seems reasonable to say that we will never know the truth. We might need a hypothesis to change people, but that doesn't mean the hypothesis will ever be scientifically validated. Certainly, it won't be validated by actions in therapy because many truths lead to results. Since we will never be sure of knowing the truth, therapy must be constructed on the basis of our best knowledge and of what is most practical. Within that framework it does not seem too audacious to discuss choosing the best therapy theory.

WHAT IS TRUTH?

A woman is brought to a therapist by her husband. He says the problem is that for many years she has been unable to leave the house alone. If she tries to go out by herself, she panics and gets terrible headaches. It is only possible for her to go out if she is escorted by her husband or her mother. She says she can't help herself. The husband says he is tired of this problem since he must work all day and also run all the errands, do the shopping, confer with the children's teachers, and so on.

Why can't this woman leave the house alone? Suppose we set out to learn the truth. It will be an unending search biased by the way we describe the problem—we hypothesize within a theoretical framework.

86

Each idea we come up with is a new perspective leading to more hypotheses or even to an alternate theoretical framework, yet none of these can be scientifically verified.

Let me cite a puzzling case. Neil Schiff, a colleague I have worked with for many years with many difficult cases, was referred by a pediatrician a case of a 12-year-old boy who still wet his bed. He had done so for years, and his mother had tried for years the various attempts at solutions. Schiff asked the parents a question that is often asked by a directive therapist: "Are you willing to do anything to get him over this problem?" The mother said she was willing, the father seemed less so. Schiff said, "I want you to give your son $50 every time he wets the bed." The mother agreed, but the father was less enthusiastic. The mother followed Schiff's instructions, and the boy made $150. Then he stopped wetting the bed. When the mother told the pediatrician what had been done, he called it ridiculous and said, "You don't reward a child for having a problem you want him to get over." The mother said, "I don't care, he stopped wetting the bed."

Apparently, the pediatrician was thinking in terms of learning theory and positive reinforcement whereas Schiff was thinking more along the lines of the ideas offered in this book. When one investigates therapy, one is often puzzled by the premises of the therapist. Whereas researchers have the leisure to explore all the possibilities associated with each variable they choose to study, clinicians do not have this option. Studying the variables in the therapy context makes the real truth more difficult to find, even if it does exist.

While therapists may hypothesize, they must act to help their clients; researchers, on the other hand, can follow wherever their thoughts may lead them. A therapist must have a theory that leads to interventions that will bring about change in the client as promptly and painlessly as possible. Can researchers ever offer therapists the truth about the cause of a particular symptom? They haven't yet, and therapists can't wait another generation. Let's give up the idea that we will find the truth, and let's choose the best theory for a therapist whose task is to bring about change in a client.

Human beings have no choice but to make hypotheses and create theories. Apparently, it is our nature to hypothesize about why other people do what they do. This is not a choice but a compulsion.

A THEORY FOR THERAPISTS

Therapists must theorize, but they cannot settle for any old theory—although that sometimes seems to happen. The hypotheses selected must be used to build a theory that is a guide to bringing about change in clients. The theory must have other characteristics as well.

First of all, the theory must give hope to therapist and client. Persons in distress must have a therapist who believes that positive change is possible for them and who demonstrates this to them. Theories of incurability are not welcome in therapy (although sometimes they are a relief to a failing therapist). Next, the theory should guide therapy to success in the majority of cases. Clients should have better outcomes than those who undergo spontaneous remission or those in waiting- list control groups.

As much as possible, the theory should describe people and problems in everyday language. Such language guides a therapist to implement change in a client's life and is not the language of diagnostic categories. For example, a supervisor who teaches trainees that the woman who can't leave her house alone should be described as agoraphobic is just being old-fashioned. Describing her as a woman who is unable or unwilling to leave the house alone defines the problem and indicates what needs to be done.

Rather than simply present the best therapy theory here, allow me to demonstrate a teaching approach by discussing the decisions therapists of any school must make. Trainees need to be involved in choosing an approach and thinking it through with the guidance of the supervisor, who, of course, hopes that in facing these decisions trainees will be led logically to the discovery that his or her views are the best ones. The supervisor must point out that trainees have no choice about whether or not to make certain decisions: When a client appears, they must take a position on certain variables whether they like it or not.

The Variables of Therapy

As in the example of the woman who couldn't leave the house alone, therapists are always faced with the question of how many people to include in defining a problem. One's hypothesis about the nature of the problem is based on the number of persons in the description of it: one person, two person, three people, or more.

A One-Person Problem

A therapist who thinks in terms of problems involving only one person would describe the problem of the woman who couldn't leave the house unaccompanied as an individual one. Such a therapist might offer the following descriptive statement: "She can't leave the house alone without becoming overcome with fear." A second hypothesis arises when the therapist proposes that the client is "afraid" to leave the house. Not only has the matter been defined as a one-person problem, but the cause of the woman's behavior has been identified as fear. A hypothesis of fear then leads to the many ideas of therapy about fear and anxiety. With this view, one is inevitably led to concentrate on the woman's inner processes because no other person is in the picture. A psychodynamicist might suggest that the woman has unconscious impulses that frighten her whenever she tries to leave the house, that is, that she panics and can't leave the house, because there are unconscious consequences to doing so. There are approximately 32,480 books on psychodynamic theory, most of them dealing with some aspect of fear. Supervisors can easily find reading lists for trainees.

There is also the popularity of cognitive theory, which includes most of the hypotheses of psychodynamic therapy but struggles to be more rational with irrational problems. There are many publications expressing this approach also. In addition, this view is supported by the literature of the behavior therapists who specialize in fear and anxiety. Trainees who take the individual view have a lot of company. Everyone, including the general public, knows how to think about a person's inner nature. The concept is at least 3,000 years old, dating back to the Greeks who explored and categorized individual character. Most trainees have supervisors who teach these ideas, just as their supervisors had supervisors who taught them. This book adds to the sparse literature that argues that therapists would be more successful if they dropped the individual as the unit addressed in therapy. The range of possible interventions is too limited.

How About a Dyad?

What if we broadened our view by placing two people in the picture? With regard to our sample case we might say, for example, "This is a woman whose husband reacts negatively if she leaves the house by herself." We are talking about the same woman, but the problem is defined differently, with a different hypothesis built into the description. We don't have so many ideas and theories about the two-person unit—nor is it thousands of years old—but for 40 years there has been enough therapy experience with it so that a therapist has to decide whether to include the husband in the description of the therapy problem. We could hypothesize, for example, that (1) the woman can't leave the house alone because she is helping her husband; (2) the couple has a marital contract, a set of rules, that she is to be helpless and he is to be helpful; (3) the woman helps her husband by having him take care of her and feel exasperated with her, thus distracting him from his own problems and providing him with an explanation for his difficulties with her and others; or (4) there is a sequence the couple follows that involves the wife threatening to leave and the husband responding to prevent it. The hypothesis need not be the actual cause of the client's behavior, but it is an explanation that guides the therapist's in devising a plan for change. For example, the therapist can put the husband in charge of helping his wife successfully go out of the house, since he says he wants her to get over her problem. The therapist could help him guide his wife step by step as far as he could tolerate, with the therapist guiding him and helping him resolve his various problems. In this approach the husband also changes.

We could also describe the problem in our sample case as a dyadic one between the woman and her mother. For example, we could hypothesize that the woman has never really left home to establish an independent life with her husband and that her symptom requires her mother's constant involvement with her. We might also hypothesize that the woman feels she needs to occupy her mother. This hypothesis would fit a theory of a family life cycle.

A problem with the dyadic description of people is that it seems unstable. We find ourselves falling back on the one-person unit, or we shift to a larger unit. Perhaps this is why there is no systematic theory of marriage therapy. The therapist ends up exploring the spouse's motivation or enlarging the unit to include someone else, for example, a lover, a child, or the mother-in-law.

Sullivan suggested that there are two people in the room in individual therapy.[1] What the client does is in response to what the therapist does. This view was abhorrent to psychoanalysts in the 1940s because their theory had no language for two people. The analyst was said to be only a blank screen at the beginning of therapy and a projection of the client thereafter. An attempt was made to use the term "transference" as a description of the two-person unit in the therapy room, but obviously it is not. It is a description of one person's perception of a relationship, not the actual relationship.

It can be argued that the minimum perceptual unit in therapy is the dyad (and later I will suggest the triad can be thought of as the minimum perceptual unit). Just as we see an object against the background of another object, so too do we see a person in the context of another person—the observer. In our classification system we cannot have a unit

[1]Sullivan, H. S. (1947). *Conceptions of modern psychiatry*. New York: William Alanson White Psychiatric Institute.

of one except as a frame for another. As Lao Tse put it, "When we create good, we have created evil." A single unit cannot exist.

Most strategic interventions are conceived of in terms of the dyad. Perhaps that is because therapists usually discuss the relationship between client and therapist, a dyad (hypnosis has also been considered a two-person phenomenon). Many interpretations involve the client's response to the therapist. For example, the presentation of a paradox by the therapist is described as leading to a reaction in relation to the therapist. Most descriptions of marital problems are dyadic in the sense that they describe behavior between husband and wife. For example, the case of the woman who couldn't leave the house could be described in terms of the husband's reaction if she were to go out alone.

Let us give short shrift to the one-person unit, consider the dyadic unit as not quite satisfactory, and spring to the concept of a three-person unit as the object of therapy.

The Merits of the Triad

When a therapist is forced to make a decision about how many people are part of the problem in a therapy case, the most useful unit I believe, is the triad—the literature recommending this unit is at least doubling, if one counts this book. For example, when we consider the case of the woman unable to leave the house alone, we can easily hypothesize that she is in a triangle with her mother and her husband.

Let us clarify at once that we are not discussing how many people are brought into the therapy room. One is conceptualizing the situation in terms of multiple triangular units. For example, a therapist seeing a woman in individual therapy should recognize that he is triangulating her marriage. The husband is reacting to the coalition of wife and therapist, and this is true even if the therapist never meets the husband. For years, marriage therapy was done by seeing each spouse individually, an approach that made the triangle more of a problem.

Children can be described as embedded in triangles of adults, particularly those trying to help them. A child with a school problem can be caught in a struggle between mother and teacher or between principal and teacher or between mother and father. The more conflicting adult triangles, the more disturbed the child.

Trainee therapists themselves are sometimes caught in a triangle. They are triangulated between new ideas, represented by the supervisor, and the old ideas in which they were trained, represented by a former teacher.

Summary

One solution to the problem of defining the unit in therapy is to adopt a broad, flexible viewpoint that permits one to think in different units for different problems. For example, alcoholism might be thought of as an individual disease, delinquency as a triadic problem, and difficulty with an erection as a dyadic difficulty. Because of the long tradition and seductive power of individual therapy, a supervisor who tries to teach flexibility in the perception of the unit in therapy often ends up with an individual focus and less success in therapy.

Just such an outcome can be illustrated by a historic moment in the evolution of psychotherapy. Sigmund Freud reached, and published a paper on, the conclusion that his young women patients had been sexually abused. As Freud put it, talking about the psychoanalytic method:

> Hysterical symptoms are traced to their origin, which invariable proves to be an experience in the person's sexual life well adapted to produce a painful emotional reaction. Going back into the patient's life step by step, guided always by the structural connections between symptoms, memories, and associations . . . I had to realize that the same factor was at the bottom of all the cases subjected to analysis, namely, the effect of an agent that must be accepted as the specific cause of hysteria. It is indeed a memory connected with the person's sexual life, but one that presents two extremely important features. The event, the unconscious image of which the patient has retained, is a premature sexual experience with actual stimulation of the genitalia, the result of sexual abuse practiced by another person, and the period of life in which this fateful event occurs is early childhood, up to the age of eight to ten, before the child has attained sexual maturity. . . . I have been able to analyze thirteen cases of hysteria completely. . . . The experience mentioned above was not lacking in a single case; it was present either as a brutal attempt committed by an adult, or a less sudden and less repugnant seduction, having however the same result. In seven cases out of the thirteen we were dealing with a liaison between children, sexual relations between a little girl and a boy slightly older, generally her brother, who had himself been the victim of an earlier seduction. These liaisons were sometimes continued for years, up to puberty, the boy repeating upon the little girl without alteration those practices that he had himself experienced at the hand of a servant, or governess; because of this origin they were often of a disgusting kind. In some cases there had been both assaults and an infantile liaison or repeated brutal abuse. (pp. 148–149)[2]

What Freud was offering in 1896 was a family theory of neurosis. He found that in 13 out of 13 cases there had been sexual abuse in childhood. Had Freud continued with this view, he would have established family therapy. He would have had to adopt the focus of family therapists today, who must take into account not only abusers but mothers who failed to protect their children. His thinking would have become triadic and would have involved not an oedipal fantasy but real-life family behavior.

However, Freud changed his mind a short time later. He decided that the sexual abuse of these patients did not actually occur but was a false memory, a fantasy they constructed of their world. By taking that position, Freud brought the therapy field back inside the mind of the client and away from what actually happens in the social context of the family. One of the most interesting mysteries in the history of psychotherapy is why Freud reversed himself. This mystery coincides with what is now another contemporary question: How often is sexual abuse actually a false memory, including a memory created by therapist and client following a hypothesis together? To assume that a client's memory of abuse is false is to absolve family members of all blame and to free the client of any need to confront them with their abusive behavior. Today the false memory question is raised in relation to the use of hypnosis. (One wonders if Freud was using hypnosis in the period when he offered his original view.) The issue of whether sexual abuse actually happened or was a false memory had major effects on the lives of many people. It led to analysts forcing clients to deny what they knew to be true. Moreover, at one time it was routine to hospitalize a daughter if she accused her father of incest, the reasoning being that such an accusation had to be a delusion.

On the basis of what we can learn from the history of psychotherapy, it would seem sensible for the therapists to consider triadic explanations of client's problems, for this approach focuses the therapy on the real world. It also suggests a large number of possible interventions to produce a change. If one must compromise, it can be said that the triadic view can be used while still respecting the individual and dyadic possibilities for some unusual problem. To ignore the triangle causes harm by stabilizing the situation.

A major reason for the triadic choice is that thinking in triads opens up coalition theory, with all its ramifications: Only with a unit of three can one think of two against one. This way of thinking not only offers a

---

[2]Freud, S. (1959). Heredity and the aetiology of the neuroses. In E. Jones (Ed.), *International psychoanalytic library* (No. 7, Chap. 8). New York: Basic Books. (Original work published 1896)

map of family dramas but also allows therapists to think of themselves as part of the client's problem.

SHOULD THE THERAPIST
FOCUS ON THE PROBLEM?

Therapists should be taught that the most immediate decision when therapy begins, a decision that reflects their general orientation, is whether to focus on the problem presented. Or should the therapist dwell on what is behind, or around the corner from, the problem? The choice a therapist makes determines the nature of the relationship with the client. If a therapist takes a history and gathers facts, the problem is not being focused on. Constructing a genogram, the fashionable way to examine the family tree, also means not dealing immediately with what the client or family wants changed.

If their therapist focuses on the presenting symptom, clients consider themselves understood. If the therapist focuses on what is behind the symptom—or above it or below it, in the roots—clients will have to be patient until the therapist gets around to what they are paying their money to have changed. Trainees should be persuaded that an immediate focus on the problem brings the most cooperation from the client. The negative side to this approach is that the therapist always has less information than he or she desires because information is not gathered in a routine history. Unfortunately, taking a history defines therapy as a place where information about the past is gathered; after this process it is difficult to persuade the family to deal with the present and take some action.

I might mention how family therapists once worked before they learned better. When a family presented a child as being "the whole problem," the therapist would try to save the child by saying, "Well, that other child in the corner looks rather strange and your other one seems unhappy and your marriage looks pretty rocky." Then the therapist would ask the family to do something to change their organization and would find a puzzling lack of cooperation, a development that led to theories of resistance.

Since trainees don't wish to be old-fashioned, it is best to point out that contemporary therapists are different: If a family identifies one child as the whole problem, the therapist agrees with them and persuades the family to reorganize to deal with that problem child.

Long ago, therapists would say that it is not the symptom that is important but its source in the client's character and its roots. The therapists who said this didn't know how to change a symptom; they could only converse about it at length and hope that it would change. The same therapists warned that if therapy changed a symptom, a worse one would develop. That has proven to be a silly idea and is only found to happen by psychodynamicists. Such a theory can paralyze a therapist since success leads to something worse.

THE IMPORTANCE OF SEQUENCE

In regard to what is changed during therapy, a sensible view, derived from systems theory, is to assume that therapy changes sequences, not persons. Let us take the example of a stepparent in a family. Let us say that a divorced woman with children remarries not only because she is attracted to her new husband but also because she believes the children should have a father and she needs help in raising them. When the stepfather begins to assert his authority over the children, the mother reacts by saying, "You don't understand these special children. You don't know them." The stepfather withdraws, and after a while a child misbehaves. The mother then indicated to the stepfather that she needs help with the child. When he does something to discipline the child, she says something like, "You don't understand how sensitive these children are, particularly since the divorce, so let me deal with them." Later, when the child again causes trouble, she indicates to her husband that he really should take more responsibility for raising the children. This sequence can continue forever and is not limited by time or the gender of the newly introduced parent. The supervisor of this case must teach the therapist how to persuade the mother to let her new husband deal with the children in his own way since he is likely to be less severe when he is less angry at her for interfering with his attempts to deal with the children.

All family interactions are made up of sequences, and therapists must learn how to think about them and how to change them. The task is not to change the child, the mother, or the father but to change the sequences they are following. When this is done, family members' thoughts and feelings change. This idea was introduced in the 1950s. Before that time, it was thought that one selected relationships on the basis of one's ideas and feelings. Now the opposite is evident: Relationships cause one's ideas and feelings. The sequences of behaviors that cause distress can be changed, bringing more tranquility and pleasure to the family. One way to teach trainees to see sequences is to show them slow-motion videos.

There are, of course, larger sequences to be described to trainees. For example, sometimes a couple will come to therapy in a crisis, and after a few sessions they feel more tranquil and go away pleased. The therapist assumes that the therapy was successful, but 6 months later the couple returns in the midst of a new crisis. A brief therapy intervention again brings tranquility, and the couple goes off happily only to return once again in 6 months. The therapist must recognize that he or she and the couple are part of a sequence of interactions.

I recall Gregory Bateson's treatment of a family with a child who was diagnosed as schizophrenic. During therapy the father went into business for himself; this was considered a positive consequence the therapy. A few months later he went broke; this was considered a negative consequence of the therapy. Then it was learned that the father had gone into business for himself and had gone broke quite regularly over the course of several years. The cycle, then, was independent of the therapy. We are still learning which sequences are changeable and which ones merely give the illusion of change because they are part of a larger cycle.

THE IMPORTANCE OF HIERARCHY

A consequence of having a social view of psychological problems is that one must think in terms of organization rather than an individual's inner nature. We have had centuries explaining human dilemmas in terms of the individual, but only recently have we thought of the individual as part of an organization. It's easier to talk of repressed anger and low self-esteem than to describe the person's position in an organizational hierarchy, particularly one involving the therapist.

All psychological tests were created to classify individuals, and all diagnostic categories of mental disorders classify individuals. Since there are no tests that satisfactorily reveal the hierarchical complexity of a family, we must describe a person's position in the family hierarchy in anecdotal ways at this time. Consider this example of hierarchical confusion: A son threatens to harm himself, run away, or commit suicide, thus causing his parents to give in to him on an issue. In other words, he puts himself in charge of the parents in terms of determining what is to happen in the family. Problem children tend to determine what happens in families, which makes for hierarchical difficulties.

There are many complex hierarchies and networks, but the simple hierarchy of a family in treatment is sufficient for supervisors to teach trainee therapists. At the top of the hierarchy are the experts who are called upon for help by the family. Then there are grandparents, parents, and children (who have their own hierarchical order). As in any organization, there are status and power differences between members.

There is also a hierarchy among therapists in an organization or system. Since their colleagues have power, therapists must learn to collaborate with them and take their power seriously, just as they must learn to take into account the status of each family member. In this day of court-ordered therapy, clinicians can find that members of a client family have disappeared into custody without their approval. Similarly, a family member can be medicated or placed in psychiatric custody despite the therapist's objections. A first step with a client is to learn whether other therapists are involved and, if so, the extent of their power and influence on the client. A trainee can be taught to talk with the colleagues involved in his or her case in ways that achieve the desired ends. What is important is to be respectful and interested in one's colleagues' views. To war with a colleague over a client is foolish—and hard on a client.

There is a problem when a family with members in individual therapy come to family therapy or when partners come for couple therapy and one of them is in individual therapy. Let me present a common problem: A wife is in individual therapy, and at a certain point she and her therapist decide that she also needs couple therapy. Sometimes this occurs when the therapist finds that not much is happening in therapy and wants to liven it up. Instead of conducting couple therapy in his or her own office, the therapist refers the couple to someone else. When a marital therapist accepts them for treatment, the wife has new things to talk about to her individual therapist. The husband, however, has no one else to talk to, so he seeks an individual therapist for himself. Then the couple drops out of marriage therapy. It seems obvious that in such a situation the marital therapist should ask the individual therapist to suspend or terminate treatment while the couple is seen in marriage therapy. Then the marriage therapist is in charge and is not an adjunct to an individual therapist who may be working with the client differently.

Obviously, therapists must learn how to include or exclude colleagues gracefully. Sometimes colleagues who have the view that more therapy is always better encourage everyone in a family to be in therapy separately and together. Such therapists are not thinking organizationally. It is sometimes helpful to supervise trainees as they talk on the telephone with colleagues to try to win their cooperation. Supervisors who talk about colleagues and other mental health professionals with respect set a model for trainees of the attitude necessary for successful collaboration with other professionals on a case.

A primary aspect of hierarchy is the power of the therapist to give power. The therapist is capable of a kind of laying on of hands in the sense that the family member he or she listens to most respectfully rises in the family hierarchy. Let me give an example of the discovery of this power by a trainee I'll call Gerald: I was behind the one-way mirror supervising

Gerald with a family made up of a mother, father, and delinquent teenage son. I observed Gerald for a while, and then I called him out of the room. "I'm supposed to be supervising you," I said, "and I don't know what you're doing. What is your plan?" "Just watch, and you'll see," he replied. I watched a while and called him out of the room again, saying I had watched and still didn't know what he was doing. Gerald said, "I'm nudging the father." He added, "The mother has had the problems of this kid, and father was out of it. I think he should take over the problem, and so I'm building him up." "How are you doing that?" I asked. "Well," said Gerald, "when the father speaks, I pay a lot of attention to him. When mother and son speak, I don't pay them so much attention. You can see father rising." He went back in the room and, sure enough, I could see the father's status rising in the room. Mother and son paid more and more attention to him, just as the therapist did.

It is because of this capacity of the therapist to empower family members that the concept of hierarchy becomes so important, and a trainee with only an individual view cannot appreciate this. If the therapist joins an adolescent against the parents, he or she is giving the adolescent power, although the therapist might only think he or she is showing concern and sympathy. Whomever the therapist listens to most attentively gains power and status within the family. In fact, when a family first arrives in the therapist's office, the therapist's act of choosing one member to describe the problem to him or her automatically designates that person as the authority on why the family is there. Therapists can also inadvertently empower adolescents by focusing on them to improve their self-esteem.

Let's say the therapist wishes to empower a parent who has an out-of-control child. The therapist must deal with the parent in terms of hierarchy from the moment the family enters the therapy room. If, for example, a single mother arrives with her mother, with whom she lives, the therapist can assume the two women have an authority problem in relation to a problem child. What relationship the therapist wishes them to have with the child will be influenced by the therapist's behavior. (The goal is usually to have mother take care of her child and have grandmother act as an adviser and help with child care.)

Grandparents are higher in the hierarchy than parents in some cultures and not in others. With Asian families one can expect the grandparents to have more power than the grandparents in the average family in the United States, where grandparents are often set aside—unless they have financial power or are needed for child care. When a couple quarrels continually and is unable to resolve issues, there is often a grandparent involved in their marriage in an unhelpful way. These days many parents who were substance abusers have had their children taken away from them and given to grandparents. When the parents try to get their children back, there are often objections from the grandparents. The court has given the grandparents power, and parents have a problem reclaiming their children. The therapist is often called on for an opinion on who should care for the child. This can be a heavy responsibility since one is being asked to predict whether a parent will relapse.

THE IMPORTANCE OF MOTIVATION

A primary variable a therapist must take a position on is why people do what they do. This is probably more important than how the therapist views hierarchy or sequence or whether or not the therapist focuses on the client's problem. We have to make hypotheses about what motivates people. If a woman yells at her husband knowing this will cause him to treat her worse, we must explain this irrational act. If a boy cuts his wrists, we must have an explanation for this astonishing behavior. It is on the question of why people do what they do that therapists most often take sides. Often the supervisor has to shift a trainee's entire perspective on a client's motivation during therapy. (A therapist may have one explanation for the behavior of a person in the therapy room and quite a different one for that person as a citizen on the street.)

The classic motivation taught to almost all supervisors, and therefore to their trainees, is the concept of the negative unconscious, which means that people do what they do because of anger, hostility, greed, lust, or any of the other deadly sins. One has only to pose a case to the average clinician to hear an unsavory explanation of the client's unconscious motivation. Unfortunately, one may hear the same from a supervisor. If one asks such a supervisor why he or she doesn't advise trainees to follow their impulses in therapy sessions, the supervisor who believes in the evil unconscious will say, "My God! Heaven knows *what* they might do if they followed their impulses!" Note that it is assumed that the impulse would be an unfortunate one. Yet if therapists cannot trust their impulses, what sort of decisions can they make?

A therapist's perspective on the unconscious becomes evident in the first therapy interview. If he or she explores all the awful things the client has thought of and done, it is on the assumption that the negative ideas must come out if there is to be a cure. That is, such a therapist believes that getting clients to express awful ideas within themselves will free them from those ideas. Such an exercise can also be depressing. On the other hand, a therapist who views the client's problem in terms of what has been positive about the client's experience and discusses what attempts the client has made to solve the problem thinks in terms of a positive unconscious.

It is best to assume that a client in therapy (though not necessarily a person in some other social context) does what he or she does for a positive purpose. For example, if a wife is given to yelling at her husband, a positive unconscious view is that she is helping him in some way. One may notice, for example, that when she doesn't yell at him, he drifts away, as if he's in a depression. When she yells at him, he becomes angry. He knows what is wrong—it is her. She is pulling him together, and so helping him, at a cost to herself. A therapist who adopts this view will have a positive view about the woman rather than thinking of her as a hostile creature. Therapists work best with a positive view of their clients.

Implicit in systems theory is the idea that each person in the system stabilizes the system and that having a symptom is a way of maintaining the stability. A system is self-corrective, and correction comes from the interactions between the individuals. A system might be miserable, but it's stable. If it begins to break up, some action takes place to prevent this. For example, when parents are about to divorce, an adolescent might take some extreme action, like attempting suicide. If a man has a sexual performance problem, his wife may develop sexual inhibitions to help him. The members of the organization or system pull together to deal with the crisis, and in the process the system stabilizes. If what makes the system unstable is not resolved, the process might repeat itself in a systematic way.

Given this way of thinking, the best theory of motivation is that people help each other—even by hitting each other. This explanation helps therapists in a variety of ways. For one thing, it gives them a positive view of the client as a cohelper. Unfortunately, clients can help other family members by harming themselves. Once a therapist understands this, it's possible for him or her to think of ways clients might help others without harming themselves. For example, if a therapist recognizes that a daughter might be helping a depressed father by giving him the task of trying to stop her from taking dope, the therapist can arrange for her to help him in a positive way. In one case, father and daughter went on a joint diet and exercise program, which mother supervised. When therapists learn to view a client's problem as involving more than one person, they begin to think of symptoms not only as attempts to communicate with others but also as helpful in motive.

IS THE BEST THEORY OBVIOUS?

From our examination of the aforementioned variables, which every therapist must take a position on, it's clear that supervisors must select the correct ones to enable their trainees to do successful therapy. It seems apparent that the theory chosen should lead to a positive view of clients by the trainee. The motivations of clients should be thought of as helpful, not vengeful or harmful. Trainees should be taught to focus on the presenting problem, since that is what people want solved, and supervisors need to know how to intervene to solve presenting problems.

The number of people defined as part of the problem should be at least three. The triangular unit allows therapists to think in terms of coalition theory. Such a view helps the therapist understand organizational problems and create interventions. One can always find three people involved with the problem, particularly if the clinician is included. When a case involves a child, a triangular unit often includes a grandparent who sides with the child against the parents and from whom the child draws power, or the therapist who may serve the same function. When there are cross-generational coalitions, as when someone higher in the generational hierarchy joins someone lower against someone in the middle, there can be confusion, difficulty, and symptoms.

It is evident that therapists need to think in terms of hierarchy and also that they can't think that way with an individual view. One can discuss how the person thinks about hierarchical position, but not what position each person actually has. Hierarchy can be discussed with the trainee in broad terms or in specific detail, depending on the supervisor's interests. That is, one can think of hierarchy when planning the entire trajectory of a case, or one can consider it in terms of details, like which family member should be asked first what the problem is. Obviously, therapists have the power to give power, appropriately or inappropriately. A therapist who prefers to avoid thinking in terms of power and hierarchy must recognize that the mere act of attempting to avoid power in itself leads to a response from the client.

ILLUSTRATIVE EXAMPLES

In the contemporary view of therapy it is taken for granted that a diagnosis requires a therapy intervention. Theory comes out of action. If therapists ask their clients questions, they get rather different information than if they direct their clients to do something and then observe their reaction. A therapist sitting behind the couch gets information about a family that is quite different from what a therapist who is sitting with the family gets. Neither therapist gets truer information than the other; what they learn is simply different because of the different therapeutic contexts. If a therapist directs a client, the client's reaction indicates the diagnosis that's important for therapy.

Let me offer a historical turning point in anecdotal form. In the 1960s Edoardo Weiss, a prominent psychoanalyst, published a book called *Agoraphobia in the Light of Ego Psychology,*[3] a presentation of the analyses of women unable to leave the house alone. Reporting on a case that failed, Weiss acknowledges that psychoanalysis often goes on for years with an agoraphobic and that sometimes the person is never changed. One might then expect Weiss to write, "Therefore, we must find some other form of therapy for these women in distress." He does not. Instead, he admits that his next case was similar, and he proceeds to report another case for which he used the therapy approach that had always failed before. (At that time psychoanalysts were failing regularly, yet they never considered changing their approach. For them, the method used must continue to be used, no matter what. In fact, this attitude is still true of the analytic societies in large cities.)

At that same time, a number of therapists were beginning to try out new approaches to replace the ones that consistently ended in failure. With a new approach, new data about women diagnosed as agoraphobic appeared. When I was in practice at that time, I did therapy with a sample of wives who could not leave the house alone. Let me describe an intervention I made that brought out a new way of thinking about the problem.

A man brought his housebound wife to me. She could only go out of the house with him or her mother. He wanted her changed. I saw the couple together, and I told them I was going to ask them to do something they might think was silly. I told the husband that I wanted him to tell his wife the next morning as he left for work to stay home. He knew she wouldn't be going out, but I wanted him to tell her that anyway, and I wanted him to do so every morning until I saw them the following week. The couple seemed amused by this suggestion, and the next morning when the husband told his wife to stay home, they both laughed. The second morning it was not so funny. The third morning after he told her to stay home, the wife went out to the local grocery store alone for the first time in 7 years. In the next interview I had a very upset husband who was worried about where his wife would go and whom she would go with if she started going out alone. The wife acknowledged that she often stated that if she could leave the house she would leave with her suitcase in her hand.

This kind of reaction reveals a structure that might never have become apparent if one had talked with the woman alone about her fears and her past traumas. Therapists who think in triads find unexpected motives in their clients, and in a case like this they may find that a threat of separation has been activated because of their therapy intervention. It is not recommended here that this is the best way to do therapy with such

[3]Weiss, E. (1964). *Agoraphobia in the light of ego psychology.* New York: Grune & Stratton.

a case; I am presenting this case, which involves a reaction to a paradoxical intervention, as an example of an approach that was tried as an alternative to analytic treatment, which has proven unsuccessful in such cases. The actual result in the case presented here was a confrontation. It would have been more desirable to work with the husband toward helping his wife go out in such a way that these issues could have been resolved without being openly confronted. Therapists must decide about confrontation in advance and anticipate what might happen to a marriage if it occurs.

We might differ in our responses to problem situations and on what theories to select to guide our psychotherapeutic efforts, but let us all agree that the worst theory ever devised for clinical work is the theory of repression. This concept has required those who believe in it to think of themselves with awful things repressed inside. It has forced several generations of therapists to make interpretations about unpleasant internal elements and waste everyone's time asking people how they feel. The notion of repression has been imposed upon the general public as well as on clinicians. It is so seductive a theory that probably it will take a national campaign by clinicians to banish it so that we can have sensible views of human beings once again.

7

CONTROVERSIAL ISSUES

Tolerance shapes the world of therapists because they must deal with unusual, difficult people in out-of-the-ordinary situations. Therapists do not seek trouble for themselves but can find themselves in it. Controversial issues have to be dealt with. As with an oil well spurting from the ground, something must be done or there is a mess. Ignoring issues cannot continue indefinitely; therapists and their supervisors must take a position on both old and new ideas, even controversial ones. The social context, it is now being said, determines the choices people make and affects their decisions. Is this always so? This in itself is one of the controversies! I can remember a bright social worker saying, "You're disappearing the individual if you say that motivation is in the social system." Gregory Bateson was even more extreme: He said the mind is outside of the person.

Therapists make decisions when choosing a theory, as they believe. Or are therapists themselves programmed by the social situation, as systems theory suggests? If the latter is so, it's important to get a therapy job in the right place. Yet how can we believe that a job will determine our ideas? Surely, therapists working in inpatient units have the same theories as therapists in private practice. Or do they? What about this book? Does it guide the reader to an independent decision based on sound arguments? Or does it influence the reader largely because it expresses the social context of a fashionable contemporary theory? Let's assume that everyone these days can boldly face issues, even if the opinions are unpopular, and proceed at once to some of the most troublesome new ideas.

IS THERAPY AN EDUCATIONAL PROCESS?

With the realization that people in therapy are motivated by their organizational position, the question of learning and education rises in new forms. If parents are mishandling a problem child, should the therapist educate them in child-rearing practices? Or should a therapist assume there are organizational problems and that when those are resolved, the parents will rear their child differently?

The primary approach of almost all schools of therapy has been educational. What the therapist teaches a client varies enormously, but the fact that the client needs to be educated seems to be taken for granted. Psychodynamic therapists, for example, educate clients about their unconscious constructs and how their present is related to their past. Conditioning therapists educate clients about reinforcements and teach one of the various learning theories. Cognitive therapists will often teach clients with a fear of going into an elevator what was the traumatic cause as well as ways to conquer such a fear. (Is this teaching them something they don't know or teaching them something they already know to motivate them to get into the elevator and lose the fear?) Marriage therapists point out to couples how they are provoking each other and causing bad feelings or how their behavior is a reflection of the ways their own parents behaved ("Your father hit your mother, and so you hit your wife").

Educating parents in how to parent children is now an industry. Many therapists seem to think they know how to teach people to raise normal children. When a therapist educates a client, the premise is that the person lacks knowledge about something or does not know how to behave. Therapists who accept the function of teaching clients assume that their behavior is a matter of individual choice and that clients will change their behaviors when they are properly educated, even those behaviors they at first say they cannot help.

The discovery that motivation lies in the social context suggests that a person responding to a system has little room for choice. I recall thinking that as an outsider I did not have to think like an insider. Then I realized, I was required to think like an outsider. Although most of us prefer to believe we make individual decisions, it can still be argued that the system determines our behavior and therefore our thoughts and feelings. What of those systems-oriented therapists who educate clients in how they are helplessly responsive to a system? Their premise must be that once clients are educated, they will rise above the system and thus acquire free choice to respond differently.

Therapists who educate their clients often don't like to admit that it's part of their job. They're concerned that such an admission implies that they believe they're wiser than the clients. In truth, it depends on the area of knowledge. One would need to compare the education of the therapist with that of the client to see if the therapist's knowledge is superior in all areas of learning. Or at least in what is relevant to the client's problems. So what is it that therapists should teach clients? Do the followers of different schools of thought agree on what to teach a client who is compulsively throwing up? Let's approach this issue in terms of how to avoid harm, which of course, is of concern to all therapists.

SHOULD THE THERAPIST EDUCATE THE CLIENT?

Therapy was born among people who were educated in universities and revered knowledge. One recognizes the influence of academia on therapists if one trains some who are not college educated. The latter don't seem to assume that if people understand themselves, change will automatically occur (less educated people have other biases but not that one). The more educated therapists are, the more difficult it is to prevent them from attempting to teach their clients and making interpretations about their clients' motivations.

Let's examine a major mistake that occurs when therapists try to educate clients: It's a difficult task for supervisors to prevent therapists from pointing out to their clients what they already know. Doing so is patronizing and raises resistance. For example, a trainee therapist might say to a mother, "Have you noticed that you are overprotective of your child?" This can be said with good intentions, yet it creates a problem. If it's not true, the mother will think the therapist is dumb. What is more likely with such mothers is that they know they're overprotective. Their problem is that they can't stop it; that's one reason they sought therapy. They don't need their nose rubbed in their problem. The therapist who makes such an interpretation apparently assumes that if such a mother realizes she's overprotective, she'll stop being that way. Why else would the therapist make such a comment? Not only is it patronizing and foolish to make such a comment to a mother, but it creates a problem in the relationship. The mother might not tell the therapist outright what she thinks of the comment, but at some point in the therapy when the therapist asks her to do something, she'll ignore the directive and refuse to cooperate. The therapist is then likely to consider her resistant and in need of more education. It has been estimated that 78% of the interpretations therapists make to clients are attempts to educate them in something they already know. For example, a therapist might attempt to teach a man who has a phobia about elevators that if he gets into one without feeling afraid, he'll erase the phobia; the client has probably suspected this all along.

Often the work of a therapist is empowering parents when children are a problem. The hierarchical task is to build the parents up and have them respected by the children. Yet each act of educating parents carries with it the accusation that they don't know what they're doing; otherwise, the therapist wouldn't be educating them. "You must be consistent with children," says the 22-year-old unmarried psychologist to the 40-year-old parents. "I am but my husband isn't," responds the wife. "But you must both be consistent," says the therapist. Is this education? Or is it the creation of guilt for doing what they cannot stop doing because of their troubled relationship? Isn't the problem the organization of the family system, not ignorance? What the astute reader has noticed is that supervisors have the same problem with respect to trainees. If they educate the trainees not to educate clients, they're doing exactly what they're advising the trainee not to do. How can supervisors stop trainees from making educational interpretations about what clients already know? The problem is how to change the social context so that trainees don't try to educate to bring about therapeutic change. The following case summaries illustrate these points.

Sample Case 1

A woman brought her 12-year-old son to therapy and explained that he was "limited" (whether he was retarded was unclear). She said her husband had died a few months earlier, leaving her with the burden of raising their son. To protect the boy she walked him to school, she volunteered for playground duty at lunchtime so that she could keep an eye on him, and walked him home from school. She never let him out of the house by himself. Now here was a woman, it seems, who needed to be educated in child rearing and taught that she was overprotective, that the boy needed more freedom and responsibility, and even that many of his problems were caused by her limiting his range of behavior. After such an educational discussion by a supposed expert in child rearing, the woman would probably have felt awful about the way she was raising her child. She would conclude that she had harmed him by her overprotectiveness. If she had felt too awful or angry or upset with the therapist, the boy would probably have made trouble to help her so that she could point out to the therapist that it was the boy, not she, who had the problem. A therapist who believes that self-understanding is the goal for clients would say that it was essential for this woman to realize how bad she was at child rearing, even if this realization was upsetting to her.

The therapist in the case, Peter Urquhart, one of our community-based therapists, talked to the woman and the boy for an hour. At no point did he suggest to the mother in any way that she was overprotective. Following the supervisory plan, he told the woman that she would have to get ready for a change in her son, that more is expected from a 13-year-old than from a younger boy, and that he would have to take care of himself out in the world someday. Urquhart indicated that there was no rush about this change, and he asked the woman if she would let the boy play in the street after school right in front of their house, where she could watch him from the front porch to protect him. She agreed to this. Then he had her watch the boy walk to the corner and back so that he could learn to be out in the neighborhood with the other kids. She agreed to that. Within 3 weeks the boy was shooting baskets at the local playground and the mother had a part-time job. At no point did the therapist criticize in the name of education the way this woman was raising her son.

There was another interesting event in the treatment of this case. The mother said that at times she could hear the boy talking to his deceased father up in his room. This worried her. Many therapists would immediately assume a diagnostic posture and think of the boy as psychotic, but Urquhart turned to the boy and said, "What does you father say to you up in your room?" The boy replied, "He says I should have a bicycle." Urquhart asked the mother, "What about that?" The mother agreed to let the boy have a bicycle but said he could not ride it.

The next week, when she saw the therapist alone, she said that sometimes at night her deceased husband would come up the stairs and lie down in the bed beside her; then he would sigh and go away. It seems possible that the mother would not have made this confession if her therapist hadn't responded so matter-of-factly to the boy's imagined conversation with his father. Urquhart then educated this mother by saying what she already knew, namely, that lonely people sometimes see relatives when they miss them very much. The visitations ceased.

In this case the therapist had to make a choice about the goal of therapy. He had to decide if the goal of the therapy was to educate the mother about her child-rearing practices or if it was to get the boy to maximize his potential and to interest the mother in something besides the boy. How would educating the mother about her child-rearing practices have achieved that goal? She needed a son who could fulfill his potential, not an education.

Sample Case 2

Parents brought to a child guidance clinic a 4-year-old boy and his 3-year-old sister. Both children had problems. The boy screamed and yelled all the time he was out of the home, and he clung to his mother; his little sister imitated him. The parents helplessly tried to deal with the children and were obviously in conflict about how to raise them. Since I was supervising that day, and happened to be irritated with some behavior therapists who were educating mothers in a patronizing way, I wondered if it might be possible to change the children's behavior and the child-rearing practices in this family without ever explicitly teaching the mother anything about child rearing or about learning theory or about reinforcements. That was the task I gave to the therapist. I told her that she could talk to the mother about all her relationships except her relationship with the children, and that she couldn't say anything to the mother about how to raise children. The task was not an easy one because of the children's wild behavior. The husband at first declined to come for therapy, which made the task more difficult. Therapist and mother talked about her relationships with her mother and her husband, but did not discuss the children. After a few sessions the children were able to be separate from their mother enough to play in the waiting room while the mother talked in the therapy room. They also stopped yelling.

As the children's behavior improved, a conflict arose in the marriage. The husband, apparently feeling more neglected by the wife, said they could not afford therapy anymore. During a therapy session the wife angrily stated that she had put up with too much from her husband, a complaint she had not previously voiced. The therapist then saw the husband alone and encouraged him to do more socializing with his wife so that they could get some enjoyment out of life. Attending therapy sessions together, the husband and wife worked out their difficulties, and the children became well behaved enough to be accepted in nursery school.

At no point in her handling of this case did the therapist educate the mother about parenting, although the mother apparently thought that this was what the therapist was doing, since she told someone that at the guidance clinic where they were guiding her in how to raise children. During the therapy the woman talked about how she needed to be consistent with her children, how she and her husband needed to back each other up, how she needed her mother to advise her but not to take over, how children need love and attention, and so on. These are among the ideas therapists often teach to mothers, and this mother seemed to know them without being taught.

Both the supervisor and the therapist for this case assumed that the parents and children were caught up in an unfortunate organizational sequence. When that was changed by directives, the children changed. The assumption, then, proved to be correct.

In general, therapists should assume that parents know how to parent. There is considerable knowledge about child rearing available from relatives, friends, neighbors, television, magazines, and so on. If parents are doing it badly, it is probably their family system that is in trouble, not the parents' mental processes. The goal is to put the knowledge into effect. One can suggest to parents certain child rearing techniques as a way of motivating them to act in special ways, but that doesn't mean they don't know how to parent to start with. Some therapists might think that educational interventions are always appropriate, but if parents feel patronized or blamed as inadequate, they suffer and resist further therapeutic efforts. On the other hand, to educate parents in child rearing because they request it is courteous. However, believing that education is the cause of change can be naive.

Sample Case 3

Let me give an example of a different kind of education. I was strolling down a hall in the clinic when a Hispanic trainee stopped me and said, "I just got a 13-year-old boy out of bed with his mother. He had always slept with her." The trainee looked pleased with his success. I knew that many therapists would educate a mother about how she might be lonely or have feelings for her son that would make her want to sleep with him. If they did not say this directly, they would imply it, believing that the woman needed to be educated as a parent. The problem is that if the mother is educated about having a desire to sleep with her son, she would feel she had done wrong. What therapist wants that? I asked the trainee, "Well, how did you do it?" He replied, "I thought he was too old to be sleeping with his mother, so I thought about how to change that. I saw the mother alone and said I wanted to suggest something to her privately. I said that her boy was now 13 years old and that in the mornings he would be getting erections and would be very embarrassed if he gets an erection in the presence of his mother. I said I thought it might be better if he sleeps by himself. She said that I was right about that, that he would get embarrassed. She had even noticed that he turned away from her in the morning. Now she has him sleeping elsewhere."

I thought that this trainee's approach was a sensible form of education designed to fit the therapy rule that clients should never be made to feel more unhappy or guilty that they already feel.

Conclusions

There seems to be some confusion about learning and education. If a man builds a bridge and it falls down, someone can educate him about how to build a better bridge. He will benefit from that knowledge in his next attempt at bridge building. However, if that man has a troubled relationship with a woman, a therapist educating him about improving the relationship does not necessarily make the man's life more tranquil. Educating people about their social or animate environment does not seem to lead to success as surely as educating them about the physical environment. In other words, as a colleague of mine said, "If you kick a stone, you can compute the distance and trajectory of that stone. If you kick a dog, your predictions are not as valid." The same is true of educating clients about their personal relationships: Live objects are different from bridges.

What rule, then, should we follow on educating clients? I suggest the following guidelines:

1. Since many young people today believe that life is changing so fast they can't trust information from their elders, they often seek out a contemporary expert. If a therapist is an expert in some area, he or she should certainly educate the client in the sense of providing information that is sought. For example, teaching a client about AIDS, if one knows that subject well, is certainly reasonable. This is different from telling a mother she's raising her children poorly and expecting this information to transform her.

2. If a therapist cannot refrain from interpreting and educating, he or she should make sure the ideas presented are positive.

3. If a therapist cannot stop being an educator, he or she should modify this compulsion by restraining any attempt to educate clients about their motives.

DOES THE PAST CAUSE THE PRESENT?

Up until the middle of this century it was taken for granted in the field of psychotherapy that events from the past cause what happens in the present. A symptom—such as a phobia, a compulsion, or anxiety—was considered maladaptive or inappropriate behavior in the present carried over from past experiences. Having a compulsion to wash one's hands was taken to mean that some past experience caused some fear that made this behavior necessary. If a man drank too much, the family in which he was raised was assumed to have been dysfunctional. This idea that a person helplessly responds to past stimuli, most of them unconscious, influenced thinking both in and outside the field of psychotherapy. Thus, if a woman today is sexually inhibited, she often believes that she must have suffered sexual abuse as a child even if she can't remember it.

I recall in the 1950s talking to a psychiatric resident on the grounds of a hospital. He was telling me about a young man he was seeing in therapy. I asked if the young man was married. The resident didn't know. Yet he had been doing therapy with the young man several times a week for 6 months. The resident's lack of information about the client's present situation was not at all surprising to me; some of us at that time were helping psychotics live through the oral phase of being infants. We didn't notice that being in the hospital was part of their problem. We believed that their childhood was their problem, and were seeking the truth about early influences. We were only just beginning to accept the patient's present context as relevant, a context such as being confined in a hospital and having the family waiting at the gate.

When I conducted therapy in those days with clients diagnosed as schizophrenic, I interviewed them an hour a day, 5 days a week, for years. That was how therapy was done. It was after years of treating a young man that I began to realize that his problem was being in the hospital. He had been locked up for 15 years; when I took him out to a restaurant, he did not know how to order from a menu. Yet he was supposed to be cured while living in the hospital, and it was assumed that he would then be able to go forth and make his living. His current social context was not considered relevant.

Contemporary therapists might not realize how embedded in theory we were in those days. I recall doing therapy with a young man who regularly said his stomach was full of cement. He said it as if he really believed there was cement in there. He also had other delusions. As his therapist, I was thinking of his problem as being related to his fixation at the oral stage, with the cement representing mother's milk. As John Rosen put it, the future schizophrenic was sucking on a breast of stone.[1]

I consulted Milton Erickson about this case and asked him what he would do. He said, "I would visit the hospital dining hall and see how the food is. Then I would talk to him about digestion." I thought Erickson was not appreciating the power of the oral stage, then I went to the dining hall. The food was pretty awful. Then I started to talk to the patient about digestion, as Erickson had recommended, and it seemed to help.

When therapists today talk about the past causing a symptom, they are repeating what was taken for granted by two or three generations of

[1]Rosen, J. N. (1951). *Direct analysis.* New York: Grune & Stratton.

therapy supervisors. Most teachers of therapy still have that notion, which is why this issue is still controversial. The question of whether the relevance of the past is anything more than a metaphor has been raised by proponents of systems theory. The idea arose in the 1950s, that a symptom is adaptive, not maladaptive, behavior. With the argument that a symptom is an expression of the person's current situation, that is, appropriate in the social context where it occurs, it became obvious that one must change the social situation to change the symptom. This meant changing families and hospitals.

The question is whether the "cause" of a symptom is in the present or in the past? Obviously some behaviors that began in the past continue into the present, like doing arithmetic or driving a car, but what about symptomatic behaviors? Let me clarify the issue with an example. Suppose a person who is afraid to ride in elevators sees a therapist. The therapist can think of this fear as caused by a past trauma having something to do with enclosed spaces. Or the therapist can assume that the fear has some function in the present. Does avoiding the elevators benefit the person socially in some way? Or the therapist can entertain both ideas—past cause and present function— or view them as interesting but not relevant to therapy. The goal is to get the client into an elevator without fear, which might be accomplished without exploring the past or taking the current function of the symptom into consideration (a phobia can be changed without necessarily even dealing with the latter).

Educating clients and talking to them about their past can best be thought of as a courtesy procedure. Since clients have the popular belief that the past causes the present and should therefore be discussed, they often expect a therapist to teach them. Such a discussion about the past can foster a relationship that allows therapeutic intervention to make a change in the symptom. A client's expectation that the past will be discussed wins the client's cooperation in taking some action.

The confusion about the cause of symptoms has been encouraged by the way insight into the past can come about after a therapeutic change. Rather than assume that insight into the past causes change, it's better to think of change causing insight into the past. For example, I helped a taciturn man recover from headaches that had been his curse for years. According to his own hypothesis, their causes were physiological. With the help of a paradoxical directive, he recovered from the headaches. At that point he wanted to flood me with information about what in the past had caused these headaches. He needed to make sense out of getting over the problem, and he brought up hypotheses and explained them to me. It seems obvious that therapists who change people should listen politely about their insights about the past after the change has occurred. Therapists should be taught to respect insight as an aftermath of change.

WHAT ABOUT FALSE MEMORIES?

A woman who suffered from a fear of drowning, which handicapped her in various ways, sought help. She went to a therapist who hypnotized her and took her back to a previous life. In that life she saw her sister drown. It was claimed in a workshop that when she remembered that past life experience, she lost her fear of water. Another woman with a fear of water retrieved, during therapy, a memory of her sister drowning as a child in this life. Remembering that was said to relieve her fears.

Should supervisors teach trainees to take clients back to previous lives and have them recall traumas? If it relieves the symptom, why not? Is it unethical for a therapist who doesn't believe in past lives to act as though he or she does in order to treat a client who has this belief? Supervisors must take a position on whether there are past lives, whether they influence us, and whether there are such things as false memories. Those who do not believe in the existence and influence of previous lives cite the fact that some clients claim to have retrieved memories of a past life as proof that memories can be false.

The issue of false memories cannot be lightly dismissed. There are false memory situations that are complicated and seductive. Memories are fragile. Even real memories come and go, being available at some times and not at others. With hypnosis, quite early memories can be revived, but memories that are false also can be "recalled." That's one reason for not allowing testimony obtained with hypnosis in court trials. Memories brought forth in therapy are a product of the relationship between client and therapist. Depending on that relationship, there can be "real" or false memories. Memories can be influenced by hypnotic suggestion as well as by the ideology of the therapist. A past-life therapist and a psychoanalyst can each influence the person to have memories appropriate to the relationship. We must keep in mind that the theory of repression is a product of a collaboration between client and therapist.

It is a tragic situation when a daughter has a false memory, engendered by her therapist, of being sexually abused by her father, and is encouraged to confront her parents with this "truth." It is also tragic when a daughter has an accurate memory and tries to get the truth admitted and her father, with her mother's support, denies it. What position should a supervisor take when a trainee has a case in which the client claims to have a memory of sexual abuse? Supervisors should remind trainees that false memories can be produced by a therapist and his or her client. As with many other problems in the clinical situation, the influence of the therapist can be overlooked or minimized. Supervisors must make it clear that the therapist is part of the context that organizes beliefs.

One of the most difficult moments in family therapy is when one family member accuses another of abuse and the other denies it. The therapist must make his or her best estimate of what might have happened. If the "victim" has had therapy, particularly with hypnosis, that should be considered relevant in these days when therapists are focused on childhood abuses.

Supervisors must encourage tolerance towards clients on the part of trainees with respect to issues of (1) the past causing present symptoms, (2) client education, and (3) false memories. That is, therapists should learn to talk politely to clients about the past while focusing on the present, where the presenting problem is. They should politely educate clients, when this is appropriate, while assuming that directives, not education, produce changes in symptoms. They should learn that it is possible for a client to have false memories and to feel certain that they are true, and also possible for a client to doubt a true memory; clients may even insist on the validity of a memory they know is not true in order to support some ulterior motive, perhaps in relation to the parents. Generally, therapists have fewer complications if they deal with the present, not memories.

I recall an unusual videotape of a family therapy session Braulio Montalvo would show to his trainees. The videotape was of a conversation between therapist and family, by the end of which, the little girl in the family is crying and the father, encouraged by the therapist, is admitting that he is too hard on her. After showing the tape, Montalvo would ask the group of trainees to identify the person who made the little girl cry. The group always says that the father did so because he is overwhelming the daughter. Montalvo would then run the tape backward to the point where the little girl started crying, and, as it turns out, this is when the *therapist* is talking to her, unsympathetically. Yet the members of this family, the therapist in the case, and the group of trainees watching the videotape, are all confident in their memory that the father made his daughter cry. That's how easily false memories can develop.

The following vignette illustrates the dilemma of therapists. An 18-year-old was brought to a psychiatric hospital by her parents. She accused her father of having had sexual relations with her. Her mother angrily denied the possibility of such behavior. The daughter shouted that it had occurred. The father said that he didn't know if it had occurred or not, that he was drunk at the time. When seen alone, the daughter said that she had been hospitalized three times over this issue, that each time she brought up the incest charge, she had been put in the hospital (as was standard procedure 30 years ago, when it was assumed that a daughter's memory of incest constituted a delusion).

The therapeutic team was uncertain what position to take. Finally, after considerable debate, they suggested to the daughter that she drop the accusation since she was likely to be hospitalized as a result, just as she had been in the past. The daughter said angrily, "I want my father to admit it happened." She was devoting her life to winning this admission, and her parents were devoting their lives to denying it. Finally the daughter decided to drop the matter rather than go into the hospital again, a consequence the team knew they did not have the power to prevent once the staff insisted, as the team knew they would.

When discussing cases of sexual abuse with trainees, supervisors must make it clear that, at present, whatever solution is chosen is likely to be controversial and objected to. Consensus has not arrived in the field on many problems, and we must tolerate that.

Ideology and False Memories

If it can be demonstrated that clients falsely report on the past and that memories cannot be trusted, the basic ideology of the clinical field is threatened. Most theories of symptoms are based on client reports, primarily reports about the past. Personal history is the launching pad for clinical theories. The idea that clients might deliberately not tell the truth about the past can be tolerated. However, if clients truly believe in false memories and report them as fact, an entire theory of psychopathology, based on client memories, is in question. The more doctrinaire the ideology, the more vulnerable the ideologist. Obviously, psychodynamic theory is based almost entirely on people's memories, but so is the concept of posttraumatic stress disorder, allegations of past abuse, and the history of the dysfunctional family. Whatever is reported by a client about the past is accepted as evidence of what really happened.

We can increase uncertainty about the past still further by adopting systems theory. According to that theory, what a client does is caused by what other people do, not the past. A self corrective system is a correcting element in the present; the past is not relevant (except inasmuch as one might say that the system previously operated in the same way it currently operates).

If memories can be false and symptomatic behavior is a response to the present, what can the clinician do with he past? One solution a supervisor can teach is to consider the past when talking about why people do what they do and focus on the present when talking about change. Perhaps a man drinks because he was raised in a dysfunctional family; that hypothesis, however, is not related to changing him but only to an explanation of why he has the problem. Or a client might have anxiety spells as an expression of posttraumatic stress; the therapist might relieve that stress with eye movement desensitization and reprocessing (EMDR), which has nothing to do with the origin of the client's anxiety. Many of the therapeutic techniques developed to deal with phobias involve imaging as well as encouragement, and many phobia specialists now do not even inquire into the client's past, since it is not relevant to changing the person.

We live in times of revolutionary change in therapy approaches and consequently must question prerevolutionary theories. A solution for therapists who do not want to struggle with conservative colleagues is to avoid taking causal explanation so seriously, particularly those based upon the past. Supervisors can teach that the client's problems is in the present and that hypotheses about past causes can only be tentative guides for a therapist's thinking, not truths.

THE SOCIAL FUNCTIONS OF SYMPTOMS

It can be argued that symptoms serve a social function. It's also possible to say that the social function of a symptom is a creation of therapists and supervisors to guide the therapy. Let us consider, for example, a suicide threat made by an adolescent girl. This might be her way of attempting to stabilize her parents' marriage, since she might believe that her parents will stay together to help her. Some trainees are confused and think that this social explanation of a symptom is the truth. In fact, it is better to think of it as a hypothesis that guides the therapist toward an action to make a change. The hypothesis might or might not be true. In this case, the aforementioned daughter's symptom will allow the therapist to think of her in a positive way and will guide the therapist in attempts to organize the family to protect and change the daughter. It is best to think of this explanation as a hypothesis for another reason. If the therapist thinks it is a truth, he or she will be tempted to educate the parents about this truth by telling them that their daughter is helping them stabilize their marriage. Despite the therapist's good intentions, the result is that the parents will be upset by the idea that their daughter would try to kill herself to help them. The daughter's symptoms will escalate (if the hypothesis is correct), her parents and the therapist will have defeated the therapy. The result is also more suffering for the adolescent herself, in spite of the therapist's good intentions in trying to help her. The task of the therapist is to relieve her suffering as quickly as possible by making the symptom unnecessary.

We must all make hypotheses about why people do what they do. Explaining a client's actions by postulating a social function is useful and helps the therapist avoid concentrating on the client's unfortunate past. Just as directives focus the client and trainee on actions,[2] so too does the idea of a social function of a symptom guide that therapist to action. To say that a child is staying home from school to keep a depressed mother company is an interesting and helpful idea but not necessarily a truth.

SHOULD PSYCHIATRISTS
DO THERAPY OR SUPERVISE?

Anyone who has taught psychiatric residents has seen a steady decline of focus on therapy in their training. Psychiatrists have many functions, particularly in the field of research and diagnosis, and at one time they also learned a variety of therapy skills. In the past their supervisors seemed to assume they would need to know the different schools of therapy and have personal ability as therapists, especially since they would become administrators in many agencies and hospitals.

At one time not only did supervisors want residents to learn therapy, but the residents themselves were interested in learning ways to change people (especially those ways their teachers were not offering). The residents sought out different points of view on therapy. I recall a group of residents at Mount Zion Hospital in San Francisco asking me to give them a seminar on family therapy, which was new at that time. They also asked me to keep the seminar a secret from the psychiatric teaching staff, who were all psychoanalysts and wanted the residents to learn only that ideology. I was impressed with the initiative the residents took to arrange such a seminar.

With the introduction of psychotropic drugs in the late 1950s, therapy training in residency programs began to decline. Physiological causes, even mythical ones, and pharmacology became the basis of the curriculum. By the 1970s teaching residents how to do therapy required that one prevent them from discussing drugs and insist that they focus on therapy techniques to change people. As an experiment I once allowed a discussion of drugs with a group of psychiatric residents I was training with live supervision. The case under discussion involved a woman with anxiety symptoms. I let the group speculate about her diagnosis and

[2]See Haley, J. (1994). Zen and the art of therapy. In *Jay Haley on Milton Erickson*. New York: Brunner/Mazel.

recommend possible medications for her. They discussed a variety of them, citing the side effects of each medication as well as medication for those side effects. I stopped their discussion after 45 minutes. They were satisfied that they had accomplished something. Yet at the end of their discussion there was no therapeutic plan and no understanding of the social situation of the woman's anxiety or even any knowledge of whether she was married. They had not even seen the woman yet, but they competed to show their expertise in pharmacology and their knowledge of the diagnostic manual and of the mythical people described in it.

Psychiatrists have a reputation with the public of being therapists and of having the highest prestige. My experience is that, with some exceptions, they do not know the range of available therapy approaches and many have no skill in any one of them. They do not attend workshops or seminars on therapy, in contrast with members of the other mental health professions, who fill the workshop seats to learn current psychotherapeutic innovations. Their supervisors are doing them a great disservice by only teaching them organic views of psychopathology and emphasizing diagnosis rather than therapy. The result is an increasing number of psychiatrists who do not know how to do therapy and do not even understand its premises. Since they themselves have not learned how to do therapy, they believe that "talk therapy" should not be done and that medication should be used instead. When medication does not work (and this is often the case, since it does not cure people but only stabilizes them), they seek out new combinations of medication instead of questioning the biological approach to psychopathology itself.

Psychiatrists, as part of the medical profession, carry power in the clinical field. The medical lobby provides them with the needed support. Because of their increasing insistence that psychological problems are medical, an antagonism is developing between them and other therapists. A common complaint from other therapists is that psychiatrists interfere with therapy by prescribing medications without even consulting the therapist already involved with the case. Although therapists in agencies and in private practice need to have a medical consultant available, the problem is in finding a psychiatrist who will medicate in relation to the case, not in relation to some theory of incurability. Such psychiatrists are becoming more and more difficult to find. The preferred medical consultants today are family practice physicians; they, too, can medicate, but they can have a social view and do not have the prejudices of contemporary psychiatry.

More and more psychiatry is being defined as social control, an inevitable consequence of the increasing use of medication. The emphasis is on how to prevent patients from being an inconvenience to society or to their families rather than on how to help them achieve a better way of life. If a person is depressed, the first concern is what medication to give, not what might be depressing him or her. The fact that occasionally there is a person who is depressed for unknown reasons does not seem to be a sufficient excuse for drugging the patient population and not learning how to identify and resolve psychological problems.

Some of the psychotropic medications are acknowledged to be dangerous, such as the neuroleptics which can cause tardive dyskinesia, in many cases irreversibly.[3] That makes a sad future for young people since the grimacing and uncontrollable movements make it difficult to earn a living. Producing neurological damage is a serious responsibility. Equally serious is the fact that nonmedical therapists are being increasingly blocked from doing therapy with anyone diagnosed as psychotic. If a person hears voices or seems to have a delusion, he or she is taken over by medical people and drugged. Although a physiological cause for schizophrenia has been claimed for over 50 years, no scientist has yet found it. Social workers and psychologists are prevented from doing therapy with such cases by psychiatrists' proclamation that such clients are incurable and can only be stabilized. Unfortunately, after stabilization they may become incurable.

Psychiatrists who enter a therapy training program, who are rare, force supervisors to constantly deal with issues of medication, supposed physiological causes of symptoms, and the possibility of malpractice suits. This leaves little time for the subject of changing people.

I once visited a psychiatry department in the Midwest and jokingly said to the chief of psychiatry, "I understand that therapy is an elective in psychiatry now." The chief did not take this remark as a joke and replied seriously, "Oh, yes, it certainly is in our department. The residents don't have to learn how to do therapy unless they wish to." In fact it is now a problem for those psychiatrists who would prefer to do therapy to find employment where they will *not* be forced into only using medication.

Therapy programs once benefited from the presence of psychiatrists. They not only had medical contributions to make but had an attitude of responsibility that was sometimes lacking in members of other mental health professions. Psychiatrists, as part of their medical training, accept the idea of full responsibility for the client. Other professions do not teach that position. However, therapists are turning to other physicians for consultation, meaning psychiatry can be removing itself from the therapy field. At the moment, supervisors can teach that psychiatrists, social workers, and psychologists can collaborate. Social workers and psychologists pass on to the psychiatrists the cases involving depression

---

[3]A possible exception is clozapine. For readers who would like a critique of psychiatric medications, see Breggan, P. (1991). *Toxic psychiatry*. New York: St. Martin's Press.

and psychosis, and psychiatrists can refer to therapists the cases they do not wish or know how to deal with, such as those involving marital and family problems. However, this collaboration is becoming more tenuous.

WHO SHOULD DO FAMILY THERAPY?

Family therapy offers a difficult problem for both psychiatrists and psychologists. Many children and adolescents require the empowering of parents as part of therapy. The despairing parent of violent children, or those determined to be failures in life, must be encouraged to take charge and guide their offspring. If the problem is defined as a medical problem or a deep psychological problem, the parents will not take necessary action. It would be like asking them to take out their child's appendix. For parents to take charge and become involved, the problem must be defined as something in their domain. If it is diagnosed as a medical problem, they will seek a medical expert to deal with it. If it is diagnosed as a deep psychological problem, they will seek a deep psychologist.

To involve parents in helping to solve a child's problems, the parents must be persuaded that it is a behavior problem and therefore something they can act on and change. Psychiatrists and psychologists must abandon their professional diagnosis and define the problem in ordinary family terms. For example, if a child has the diagnosis of anorexia nervosa, the parents will not act to change it; they will take the child to a medical expert who knows what to do with medical problems. However, if the same child is diagnosed as one who refuses to eat, and therefore as a disciplinary problem, the parents will be willing to take action under therapeutic guidance, to make the child eat.

It is a sign of the decreasing importance of therapy to note that the three major professions traditionally spend most of their years of training learning matters hardly relevant to therapy. Psychiatrists devote years of training in medical school learning material they will never use in therapy practice. Few will even do physical examinations, unless that is part of their job on an inpatient unit of a hospital. Psychologists spend years doing research, which is of no use in therapy, although recently they have begun to use people instead of rats in their research and have begun to do outcome studies. (Now psychologists are lobbying to be allowed to medicate and hospitalize people, choosing the least therapeutic aspect of psychiatry to imitate.) Social workers, until quite recently, learned in academia what it is to be a social worker. Some social work departments have now begun to teach a variety of therapy approaches.

Members of all three professions are trained to focus on individuals: Psychiatrists diagnose a child, psychologists test the child, and both do child play therapy. The social worker sees the parents. As the focus of the field becomes therapy, members of all three professions do the same therapy and must give up much of their past training to learn new ways of working. The supervisor must judge how much emphasis should be put on a trainees professional background and how to help him or her learn to bring about changes in clients. Supervisors often meet opposition from colleagues in academia who only know past ideas about therapy and who change more slowly than therapists facing problems in the field.

WHAT ABOUT GENDER CHOICES?

Besides ideology and profession, there is another way to classify therapists: by gender. Should the gender of the therapist be a focus of supervision? Every supervisor must take a position on this.

It seems obvious that female therapists should have the same rights, salaries, positions, conditions of practice, and opportunities for advancement as males. That's a safe and easy position for a supervisor to take. Other matters, however, are more complicated.

Should the gender of the therapist be taken into account for particular problems or cases? For example, should a woman who was sexually abused as a child have a female therapist rather than a male? It could be argued that a female therapist would understand her vulnerability better. It could also be argued that a male therapist would help her "work through" those feelings she has about men as a result of this traumatic experience. Some supervisors might even consider it important to assign to this case a male therapist who had been sexually abused as a child. There are sound arguments on both sides of this issue for many types of cases. However, there is a larger issue: If one allows the idea that men are better at treating certain problems and that women are better at others, the field of therapy becomes classified by gender. This idea has huge consequences. We would soon have a diagnostic system that includes gender of therapist to be assigned to the case. Such a classification might result in the tendency for social workers to be assigned to some cases and psychologists or psychiatrists to others. It would mean that an agency would have to have sufficient therapists of each gender and profession to deal with the kinds of problems confined to each kind of therapist. This can be prevented if it is accepted policy in the field of psychotherapy that any therapist of either gender is capable of treating any symptom of any gender. It's the responsibility of the training supervisor to establish the expectation that gender, as well as ethnicity and socioeconomic levels, will not be used to classify therapists. Training should enable any therapist to treat anyone.

A more serious problem is how therapists should deal with gender issues in families. What if the wife in a family with a daughter who is presented as having a problem says that she would like to go to work but her husband won't let her? The husband agrees. A therapist with feminist views has the problem of deciding whether or not to educate the family on the rights of women. If the therapist is a trainee, the supervisor in the case must take a position on whether to encourage such didactic efforts or not. It is argued here that if the presenting problem is the daughter's behavior, that should be the focus of therapy. The therapist is in error if he or she prevents the daughter from changing by antagonizing a father whose views on the rights of women differ from the therapists. If the difference in views does not interfere with the goals of therapy, such education is reasonable. One assumes the therapist is acute enough to consider the possibility that the wife says her husband objects to her going to work because she herself is reluctant to do so and is using him as an excuse.

DOES RELIGION MATTER?

Another example clarifies the therapy issues: Sometimes therapists are religious enthusiasts and might like—in fact, are even encouraged by their religion—to proselytize. Should a therapist encourage a family to pray? This reminds me of a conversation I had with John Warkentin about a case of his. He said, "I don't think the woman would have improved if I hadn't knelt and prayed with her when she asked." "Would you have prayed with her if she hadn't asked you to?" I inquired. "Of course not," he replied. "I'm not a religious man."

The personal crusades of therapists should be subordinate to the goal of the therapeutic undertaking. The goal of therapy is to change the problems clients bring, not to convert or educate them in feminism, psychodynamic theory, or Christianity.

THE DUAL HIERARCHY

Therapists need supervisors who will help them with their prejudices about various issues, particularly the status of women. A problem for therapists is how to be fair about gender rights while also joining a family that belongs to an ethnic group that has unfortunate ideas about the equality of women and men. The revolutionary changes in women's status are certainly not worldwide. Supervisors must guide therapists to an ideological orientation that is satisfactory to their conscience and that also allows them to work with and benefit the family in therapy. In this complex situation there are one or two issues that supervisors can emphasize to help achieve objectivity.

The question of equality between a husband and wife is a special concern to us all. What should be the hierarchy in the marital dyad? There are cultures where women have no rights in marriage at all, but even in our culture there are situations that are more organizational that ethnic. For example, a young college educated couple marries and builds their relationship on equality, sharing their decisions equally. Neither has power over the other. However, everything changes when they have a child. At that point they become coleaders of a group. Hierarchy becomes an issue. They must reach agreement on who is in charge of what in relation to the child. Who will decide how the child is to be disciplined and educated? The problem is that husband and wife cannot be equal leaders when there is a group, even if that group is made up of only one child. According to the Fifth Law of Human Relations, there is no viable organization among human beings or animals that has two equal leaders. Can one imagine two equal presidents of the United States? The married couple must decide who is in charge of what in relation to the child.

The typical way couples resolve this problem, often with the help of a therapist, is to divide up the territory. One takes charge in one area and the other in another area. Traditionally, the wife takes charge as the primary child rearer, and the husband assumes responsibility for the family financial support. When the wife has a career, the husband might take over the child rearing and participates more in the home. One parent might become responsible for handling the child's extracurricular activities while the other handles school issues. The issue of who is in charge depends on the area in question, and much conflict is avoided.

There is another solution that involves pretending. This was a common solution for families for many years and still is. What happens is that one person takes charge but pretends that the other is in charge. The typical example is the wife who takes charge of the family but pretends that the husband is the boss when a specific issue is raised. That is, there is what can be called a dual hierarchy. It can be argued that there are always at least two hierarchies in any organization: an overt one and a concealed one. For a family there is a public hierarchy, in which the husband is in charge, and a private one, in which the wife determines what happens, which is the definition of being in charge. For this dual hierarchy to succeed, the wife must pretend that the husband, not she, is in charge. An example of dual hierarchy was provided years ago by Lincoln Steffens. He said that if one wants to know who is in charge in a city, one does not seek out the mayor but one asks any bellhop in any hotel who the political boss is. This is the person who covertly runs the city while everyone pretends that the public hierarchy is the only one. Of course, any complex organization has many hierarchical subsystems, but the minimum would appear to be two.

In recent years women have decided that pretending their husbands are in charge is demeaning. They're no longer willing to hold their husbands up and pretend they themselves are weak and naive. Women have protested and taken public charge in the family, thus exposing the pretense that the husband is in charge. Conflict occurs between the spouses when they either change leadership or struggle to be equal leaders—an inviable arrangement—or they divorce. A therapist can be in a position where the pretense that the husband is in charge must be supported, even when obviously he is not. Or the couple must be persuaded to acknowledge that the wife truly determines what happens in the family and that such a hierarchy is not merely a joke.

I was once recruiting normal families for a series of studies to determine whether abnormal families differed from normal ones. This project involved selecting an adolescent in high school and asking his or her family to come in for a research interview. I included in the interview the question of which member of the family was spoken to on the telephone when the family was recruited for the study, that is, which member agreed to participate. Checking a sample of 30 normal families, I found that in 27 cases the mother made a unilateral decision to bring in the family. That means she could get the father and the teenage children to go through the inconvenience of coming in without even consulting them. All those families arrived. In two cases a father who was spoken to first on the telephone said that he would have to ask his wife. In the one case in which the father made a unilateral decision for the family to participate in the study without consulting his wife and children, the family didn't show up.

I was once interested in the concept of the powerful castrating father described by Sigmund Freud. Such men didn't seem to exist anymore. I discovered a woman who had been raised in Vienna in Freud's time, and I asked her about her family. She said that in her family her father was the boss, if not a tyrant. She said, "We couldn't even sit in Daddy's chair." Curious, I asked her how her father kept everyone out of his chair. The woman said, "Oh, Daddy didn't do it. Mother forbade it and told us if we sat in Father's chair we would get pimples on our bottoms." It might be said that her mother was in charge of her father being in charge.

One curious finding I noticed in recent years is that the majority of married couples who come for therapy present the wife as being of higher status than the husband. This is quite the opposite of the view that women are being subjugated by patriarchal husbands. The wife presents the husband as being lower in status than she is because she makes more money or because she comes from a better family, according to their estimate, or because she is more educated, or more articulate, and so on. They come in as unequals. I am not suggesting here that women in our culture have more authority than men or are equal to men. I am talking about the population that seeks therapy. Sometimes the woman makes it quite explicit by bringing in her husband and saying to the therapist something like, "Do something about him." The woman wants her husband raised in status in relation to her and wishes him "to be a man." Supervisors focused on women's rights need to be developing ways to bring about this change that women seek.

The issue of hierarchy within a couple relationship is also complicated by the use of symptoms to communicate issues in the marriage. Some years ago it was noted that when a person says, "I cannot help myself," such an admission gives power to the helpless person. My first recognition of this paradox came with a case of a woman who was a compulsive hand washer. The woman complained that her husband was a tyrant; and indeed he agreed that he was in charge in the family and that he insisted on his own way. Yet there seemed to be a covert hierarchy behind this public one: The wife couldn't go shopping because she feared she would be exposed to contaminating liquids in the store. So the husband did the shopping. The wife couldn't wash the dishes because once her hands were wet, she had to keep washing them. So the husband did the dishes. He insisted on a clean house, but couldn't get his wife to accomplish this because it meant contact with cleaning materials containing toxic substances. So the husband did all the cleaning. With her symptom the wife required the husband to do all the menial work, even as she protested that he was a tyrant. The husband, of course, actually didn't get his own way about anything.

Once one recognizes that a symptom that communicates the idea "I cannot help myself" gains the person power in a relationship, one can understand why it is clearly the method of choice for those who feel powerless. When a wife is in a demeaning position, she may develop symptoms; this also happens with men when women gain more power. Symptoms are available to either gender. As women gain more actual power, we might see an increase in male symptoms, especially in the symptom that a husband "can't help" being unable to do what his wife wishes.

There is one other unworkable organization that therapists need to recognize in this day of divorce. There are many single mothers and fathers raising children. Often, when a parent is in charge of a group of children and there is no second in command, the children begin to overwhelm the parent. The children don't work out issues among themselves but always bring them to the parent, who is like the hub of a wheel with all the spokes going through him or her. This is an inviable organization. What is needed when one is leading a group is for a second in command to point out that the leader is the leader. This is why officers in the army have noncommissioned officers to support their authority. In single parent families, the overwhelmed parent needs someone else, perhaps the eldest child or a grandmother or the divorced father, to support their leadership, which then allows a functioning hierarchy instead of chaos.

Gender in relation to hierarchy is a complex process and not a simple male female problem. Couples struggling to be equal when leading a group are in difficulty. Analyzing the issue of hierarchy and structure in a family is no simple task since hierarchies are at least dual, inasmuch as what is shown to the public, including the therapist, can be different from the private hierarchy arrangement in the family.

The fact that the gender of the therapist, the supervisor and family members makes shifting coalitions likely means that gender issues in family therapy have no simple stereotyped solutions.

THE PROTECTIVE SUPERVISOR

Supervisors can be expected to protect trainees, clients, and themselves.

Protecting the Family Member

Generally, the supervisor must protect clients who are in the hands of trainees. I recall a type of protection that became evident in the 1960s. Here's an example: A 17-year-old went mad during her first semester in college. She was hospitalized, diagnosed schizophrenic, and sent to a hospital near her home. She began therapy with Don Jackson. In a family interview the father was speaking in a certain way to the daughter, and Jackson stopped him, saying, "If you continue that way, you'll get into trouble you don't need to get into." At that time, in the early 1960s, a therapist typically encouraged people to say anything because of the theory of repression. To stop a father from talking to his child was unusual. After the interview I asked Jackson why he did that. He said that the father was beginning to ask the daughter to judge him as a father, and it is incorrect for a parent to be supervised by a problem child. The therapist should prevent this. He added, "I think it's the duty of a therapist to prevent a father from making an ass of himself." That was a novel and refreshing idea at a time when we were all encouraging self-expression and total honesty in our clients.

Protecting the Trainee

It is the duty of supervisors to prevent trainees from making fools of themselves. One way to do that is to give them training in interview skills so they don't blunder or cast about helplessly for something to talk about. I recall a trained social worker once doing an interview with a family with seven or eight children. The social worker talked with the mother while the children jumped up and down, danced, fooled around, and yelled at each other. This made the therapist look awful, but she didn't know how to organize the family so that the mother and children could achieve some goal. I also remember observing a therapist who's been an elementary schoolteacher doing therapy with a family with four wild kids. In a matter of minutes the therapist, using her school background, had each of the four children sitting in a different corner of the room and drawing pictures; she then proceeded to talk to the mother and was able to bring the children into the discussion in an organized way.

Sometimes behavior in a therapy room gets out of hand, despite the skills of the trainee, and the supervisor behind the one-way mirror needs to intervene to resolve the crisis and save the trainee. For example, the supervisor might telephone the trainee in the therapy room and suggest that he or she divide the family into two groups and send one of them to the waiting room. Separating family members is often helpful when tensions are escalating.

If the therapist gets upset and is having difficulty because of some personal reaction, the supervisor can suggest some alternate behavior. However, therapists cannot always be protected from what is, admittedly, an upsetting business. They must be able to tolerate anxiety and still function well. To paraphrase Harry Truman, "If therapists can't stand the heat, they should get out of the kitchen."

VIOLENCE IN THE THERAPY ROOM

When they are threatened with actual danger and not mere anxiety, trainees must be protected. I was once supervising a supervisor with a case. As I went behind the one-way mirror to join him, we observed in the therapy room a mother and a daughter, with the therapist standing behind her chair. When I asked my colleague why the therapist was standing, I was told that she was afraid of the daughter, who had physically threatened her. I called the therapist out of the room and told her that she shouldn't have to be afraid of a client, that she should tell mother and daughter that if she was in any way threatened again, their therapy would end right then and there. The mother and daughter accepted this, and the therapist sat down and conducted her interview.

Since we were a private institute, we established a rule after that to not accept cases where there was a possibility of violence. Not long afterward a father walked in with his middle-aged son. He said that he had been told on the telephone that he could not bring his family to therapy because the son had been violent, and he wished to talk with someone about this. Marcha Ortiz, one of our supervisors, interviewed the man and his son and decided the family could be accepted. They were seen, and the son was never violent. Later, a middle-aged brother threatened violence, but the problem was resolved without any violence occurring.

SUICIDE THREATS

When difficulties arise in therapy, the supervisor must protect the client. The reason for using a one-way mirror is to enable the supervisor to see what is actually happening in the therapy room and to protect a client from a naive trainee, if necessary. However, there are situations where the trainee, too, must be protected. One of those moments arises when a client threatens suicide. Trainees should be taught to always take suicide threats seriously, even if they are casually made, particularly the threats of young people. If an adolescent threatens to kill himself or herself, this escalates the therapy situation to a different level, and the therapist is no longer dealing with the usual adolescent–parent power struggle.

Trainees should be taught that in addition to helping the adolescent who threatens suicide and attempting to solve the problem behind such a threat, they must hallucinate themselves on the witness stand responding to a prosecutor asking, "What steps did you take to save the deceased person's life?" Trainees, with the help of the supervisor, should be able to outline satisfactory steps. These include a willingness to hospitalize the adolescent even though this might cause the young person more difficulty than would a continuation of outpatient therapy. That is, once in a psychiatric ward, the client has been stigmatized, and such a stigma can compromise social relations, the client's eligibility for school admission or employment, right to drive a car, and so on. Moreover, hospitalization may encourage family members to view the young person as defective. Even so, hospitalization of an adolescent who threatens suicide may be necessary to protect trainees from being blamed for a tragedy.

If the trainee is being observed by colleagues and a supervisor behind the one-way mirror when a suicide threat is made, there can be a discussion that leads to support by a number of professionals for the therapist's decisions.

Although it apparently has not been tested in court, one of the better ways to deal with suicide threats is with the use of the family. If the parents will take responsibility, the therapist can organize the family in a "suicide watch." The problem client is never left alone but always has a family member with him or her. This protects the suicidal person and brings out many issues in the family as the members deal with the inconvenience.

COLLABORATION WITH COLLEAGUES

Supervisors need to protect trainees from the social system, including colleagues with authority of different kinds, as well as from the court system. Therapists must learn to negotiate their rights in relation to their colleagues. At times, the supervisor needs to be not only an adviser to the trainees, but a barrier between them and their fellow professionals. Sometimes trainees are attacked by colleagues for not taking the DSM-IV diagnosis seriously even though that classification was not designed for therapy and can interfere with it. Supervisors must support trainees in this struggle. Ideological issues can take the form of attacks on the trainees approach to therapy, which may be called shallow, manipulative, unethical, or improper. Supervisors in the training program need to deal with these arguments and their sources.

There are also specialists who wish to do their tasks even if it interferes with a client's therapy. For example, psychologist's colleagues can persuade a family that a child should have a battery of psychological tests. The trainee is sometimes too shy to point out that such a battery of tests identifies the child as the problem when such a conclusion may be incorrect and is of no use to a therapy approach whose emphasis is on the family's social organization. The supervisor must teach trainees to recognize the few tests that are relevant to therapy and how to prevent others that are not, even if that antagonizes psychologists who have spent years learning Rorschachs.

It is with psychiatrists that trainees often have difficulties in collaboration. When a psychiatrist refers a case, one or more family members are typically on medication. Most young therapists hesitate to ask the psychiatrists to remove or reduce the medication even if that seems important to the therapy approach. The supervisor needs to talk with the psychiatrist about this to see what can be done. A similar problem arises when a colleague refers a couple or family for therapy while continuing to see one of the family members in individual therapy. The supervisor must see if the individual therapy can be suspended for a period of time so that the focus can be on the couple or family.

Sometimes issues of collaboration reach the institutional level. Say, for example, that a trainee has a case of a woman who drinks too much and needs detox. The preferred course of action would be for a few days of detox and for therapy involving the whole family in order to get them organized to prevent future drinking by the woman. However, detox establishments have their own programs. They may want to keep the person needing detox in the hospital for a period of weeks and then in outpatient treatment for months. A trainee hesitates to buck that system and finds his or her drinking client stolen away and subjected to a less adequate approach. A supervisor might or might not be able to influence those in charge of the detox program.

INTERMINABLE THERAPY

A trainee should be taught to terminate a case when change has occurred and the presenting problem has been resolved. The client may have other problems, but if he or she doesn't wish to deal with them, there is no need. However, sometimes client and trainee become stuck together. The trainee can always find more problems the family should deal with, and the family, pleased with the results, likes the therapist and wishes to continue therapy. The task of the supervisor is to help therapist and client disengage. One way to arrange this is to schedule longer intervals between sessions as improvement takes place. During such recesses, the family becomes interested in other matters, and the trainee has other cases to occupy him or her.

Disengagement in therapy can be a serious problem. As an example, I was supervising in New York City for a period of time. The trainees were all experienced therapists, and they brought in their own cases for supervision. The case discussion began with, "I've been seeing this case for 8 years." Another therapist would say, "This is a therapy I have been doing for 9 years." I began to realize that these therapists were bringing me cases for help in disengaging from them. They could neither cure the clients nor lose them. Since the therapy we were doing was brief, in a number of these cases it took only a few sessions for the trainee to terminate successfully. After a while, the therapists began to feel embarrassed when presenting a case, and they would say, "I would rather not say how long I've been seeing this client."

Primarily, the protection of trainees involves their interaction with members of other professional worlds that have priorities different from those of therapy. Trainees can find it a handicap to their therapeutic efforts to attempt to satisfy the needs and ideologies of their colleagues in medicine, psychology, and social work. The supervisor needs to help them clarify these issues.

OTHER CONTROVERSIAL ISSUES

Supervisors must deal with other controversies in the field, including deciding whether trainee therapists should deliberately influence clients outside awareness, whether they should encourage divorce when couples are miserable, whether they should take children out of the home and place them in a foster home if parents are neglectful, whether young adults should be advised to leave their parents and never speak to them again, and whether to release a family from therapy when the presenting problem is solved but there are other obvious problems.

These controversies need not be examined here since the sensible supervisor already has assumed a correct position for each one.

8

LIVE SUPERVISION

Live supervision is defined as a supervisor watching a therapist at work and making suggestions during the action. This arrangement can take different forms. In the 19th century clinical hypnosis was taught by having a trainee observe a teacher at work with a client, followed by the teacher observing the trainee at work. The supervisor could see what happened and guide the procedure. With the use of the one-way mirror beginning in the 1950s and later video monitors, it became possible for the supervisor to observe the trainee in action while not present in the interview. There seems to have been a series of steps in the use of the one-way mirror.[1] I can recall the stages in my own development as a supervisor. In the early days we first observed a trainee therapist from behind the mirror and made no suggestions during the interview, only before and after it. We talked to the trainee afterward about what he or she should have done. Sometimes it was painful for those of us behind the mirror to watch errors being made that could have been easily corrected or avoided with a suggestion. But we had to wait until after the session to comment. In those early days it was apparently thought, perhaps as a result of the period when confidentiality was so emphasized, that a therapy session was inviolate and couldn't be intruded upon. The boundary around a therapist and client created a private interchange—even though the session was being observed through a one-way mirror.

The next step in the development of the use of the one-way mirror was to knock on the door during the interview and call the therapist out of the room to offer some suggestions. It was discovered not only that the

---

[1]In 1957 I observed Charles Fulweiler doing therapy with a family while he observed from behind a one-way mirror. After that the Bateson project installed a mirror. Cf. Haley, J., & Hoffman, L. (1968). *Techniques of family therapy.* New York: Basic Books.

therapy improved with suggestions made during the interview, but that the therapist grasped ideas better when the supervisor's suggestions were made. Therapists didn't object to the intrusion; they appreciated the guidance. After the therapist–client boundary was broken in this way, the therapist also felt at ease coming out of the room in the middle of a session to consult with the supervisor.

The next step was to have a telephone behind the mirror connected to one in the therapy room so that the supervisor could phone in suggestions. This was less disruptive than knocking on the door. An experienced trainee can pick up the telephone, hear the supervisor's suggestion, put the phone down, and go on with the interview without allowing the interruption to be a problem. In fact, with an experienced trainee, one could not determine from the conversation immediately after the call what the suggestion on the phone had been. Beginning trainees, in contrast, sometimes have such an elaborate response when the telephone lights up or rings that the supervisor hesitates to call because it is such an obvious intrusion.

A problem occurs in live supervision when the supervisor is too active on the telephone, interfering with the therapist's autonomy. At one period we put the telephone on the wall of the therapy room, so that the therapist had to walk across the room to answer it, rather than simply pick it up from the table. This was arranged to make the supervisor's call more disruptive and therefore to inhibit supervisors from calling too often. It is important that the supervisor be brief and to the point in telephone calls. He or she should think through what is to be said, condense it for brevity, and then call. The extreme version of too much intrusion is the use of the bug-in-the-ear device, which prevents the client from even knowing when a suggestion is being made. This arrangement has two problems that make it unwise: Therapists begin to have a glazed look in their eyes while trying to listen both to their supervisor and to the family, which prevents them from maintaining good contact with the family. Supervisors, for their part, end up talking too much because it's so easy for them to intrude. When there are continual suggestions in the therapist's ear, he or she becomes like a robot carrying out the supervisor's ideas.

Many variations in live supervision have been tried, including using only a microphone in the therapy room that is connected with the supervisor's audio recorder in the next room. The supervisor can't see what's happening, but at least he or she can hear what is being said and can make suggestions.

When live supervision is done correctly, there is a plan for the interview and telephone calls to occur only occasionally. They occur when the supervisor sees a way to improve the action within a plan or sees that something is being overlooked. If a revision of a therapeutic plan proves necessary, it is better to have the therapist come out of the therapy room and discuss the revision rather than try to communicate complex changes over the telephone.

These days an alternative to a one-way mirror is an inexpensive camera in the room and a monitor in another room for the supervisor to observe. With the monitor arrangement events in the therapy room don't have quite the same immediacy to the supervisor as they do with the one-way mirror, but it is adequate. There are also new opportunities with video observation. Once one realizes that the monitor can be in the next room, it is evident that it can be in the next building. In fact, it can be in another city. One can have live supervision over any geographical distance, even from one country to another. In the early 1980s I participated in live supervision from Washington, D.C., by looking at a monitor and giving suggestions talking over the telephone to a therapist in Louisiana. The technology is available with satellites to guide therapists at work worldwide.

Live supervision is valuable as a way to teach a therapist how to carry out a therapeutic plan. Often it is simply helpful to have another pair of eyes watching a case from an objective distance to assist in practical matters such as preventing a therapist from misunderstanding what someone is saying or from neglecting a family member who should be brought into the discussion. Sometimes the therapist fails to do something he or she would normally do but has forgotten for the moment and needs to be reminded. For example, in one family session a mother said she would like to talk to the therapist without her son present. The therapist went on discussing issues, apparently thinking an interview could be arranged for the mother without the son at some future time. The supervisor called and suggested that the therapist simply send the boy out of the room and listen to what the mother had to say. This was done and saved a great deal of time. As another example, a woman client was discussing her problem and mentioned that her father had sexually abused her as a child. The woman said this in such a casual way, while discussing other matters, that the therapist did not really register it. The supervisor called and suggested that the therapist ask the woman if she had ever talked to anyone about this. It turned out that she hadn't and that she was pleased to discuss it with someone for the first time.

One problem to keep in mind is the fact that the one-way mirror screens out emotions. It's sometimes difficult for a supervisor to judge how upset a client is. When suggesting that a therapist have a client do something, the supervisor sometimes meets resistance from the therapist. The question then is whether the therapist is picking up information from the client that the supervisor does not have, or whether the therapist is underestimating the client's tolerance. For example, a supervisor might suggest that the therapist discuss sexual issues with a couple, but the therapist might be reluctant. The question is: Who is it who finds this subject too sensitive at this time—the couple or the therapist? Because there is different information available to the therapist in the room than to those behind the mirror, it is helpful for a supervisor to say to the trainee something like, "I will make suggestions to you, and I want you to follow them. But keep in mind that these are suggestions. You might decide not to do something because in your judgment, being in the room with the client, it would be better not to. However, if I say you *have* to do something, than you have to do it." A speech like this clarifies for trainees that the supervisor is the teacher and authority on the case, but that they, too, have responsibility.

THE TRAINING GROUP

Supervisors can work one-on-one with a colleague or trainee or they can work with a training group behind the one-way mirror, with the trainees taking turns going in to see clients in the therapy room. The two situations are quite different. The unit when supervising a single therapist alone is the therapist and the client. The supervisor can focus on that and easily ignore distractions. There is also freedom to comment on the therapist and his or her style in both positive and critical ways because the discussion is private.

When supervising a training group, however, whatever the supervisor says is heard by the entire group. Furthermore, the supervisor isn't free to devote full attention to observing the interview but must comment to the group about what is happening and what should happen. Sometimes just speaking what he or she is thinking helps the group follow the action as the supervisor understands it. The supervisor may occasionally become so involved in observing a trainee's handling of a case that the group is forgotten. The group of trainees may observe what is occurring in the therapy room and may reach the wrong conclusion. For example, in a particular situation the supervisor might encourage a confrontation; the group may think that such confrontation should always be done instead of understanding that it is only suggested for this particular case. It's best for the supervisor to make clear to trainees what his or her point of view is so that there is not misunderstanding. When therapy sessions are videotaped, supervisors have an opportunity to go over the material at a more leisurely pace and to thus clarify the premises on which various interventions were made.

The goal with a training group is to teach both therapy technique and an understanding of human problems. The benefit of live supervision is that it provides the opportunity to discuss a particular problem at the moment the trainee therapist and the trainee group are struggling with it.

Therapists can learn in academic settings traditional ideas about human problems and can find support for those ideas in textbooks. When the therapist later does therapy and has a case involving a type of abnormality, they try to remember what they learned about it years ago in class. Live supervision offers another way of learning: Therapists learn about a problem and what to do about it simultaneously. For example, when a student learns about mental retardation in school, it is only of academic interest. When a trainee in live supervision is given a family with a mentally retarded adult son, the teaching is of quite a different kind. The trainee is eager to learn what to do about this problem and what is known about it. For example, it may be evident that the retarded person can tie his own shoes, but that he never does so because his mother is so helpful that she always does it for him. The need to maximize what the person can do then becomes evident. The trainee can see the nature of the problem as well as the family involvements in action.

When teaching therapy, not diagnosis, supervisors find that trainee therapists learn best when they view a problem in a therapy session, not during a diagnostic interview. Not only does the trainee therapist discover the nature of the problem, but the group watching the therapy session is part of the therapy process. When meeting a similar case in the future, all the trainees will have an advantage in dealing with it.

The training group is also valuable to the supervisor. During training, every type of case is brought in, and the supervisor can use the knowledge of the group to supplement what he or she knows. In a group of trainee therapists (who are functioning therapists, not beginning students) there are individuals who have extensive experience with different client problems, medications, types of colleagues, and legal situations. A good supervisor draws on the wisdom of the group. It should be clear that the supervisor is in charge and that ideas and suggestions go from the group to the supervisor and from there to the trainee therapist handling the case.

The use of the resources of the group is determined by how the group is organized. A crucial issue is the emphasis on the positive by the group. What is wanted is high group morale. The supervisor wishes to organize the group to bring out the best ideas from everyone, just as the therapist wishes to draw on the best of the client's ideas.

Have You Heard of Emile Durkheim?

In each training group of eight to ten people there is almost always one deviant. A supervisor usually has difficulty dealing with one such trainee. This is a trainee who objects to the ideas he or she came to learn, who protests a type of directive, or who asks questions that are obviously derived from another ideology. Group members tend to ostracize this person, or roll their eyes when the deviant speaks. How should the supervisor deal with such a person? Patiently. One should accept Durkheim's idea that every group must have a deviant.[2] The function of the deviant is to show the group how not to behave. The implicit rules for behavior in a group cannot be made explicit but are broken by the deviant; so then everyone knows that is not the way to behave. I recall a sales manager saying that you should never fire your worst salesman because then you would only produce another worst salesman; the group of salesman needs a worst one. Kicking out a trainee who makes difficulty can lead to the same results.

In the many training groups I have conducted I have had many deviants but only one trainee who went mad. A curious thing happened with her: She began to confuse her personal life with her client's statements. As we, observing her behind the one-way mirror, watched her treat a couple with a problem, it became evident to us that she was not responding to the clients but to ideas of her own. The husband would say, "Some people are unhappy," and the therapist would nod wisely, as if she knew he was speaking of someone she knew, and she would say something like, "We can know that is true." Then she would say something like, "Some people say they have difficulty with the car when that is not so." The wife would say, "Yes, he often has some mysterious problem, and I don't know where he is." The young therapist completed the hour with the couple, and at the end the husband thanked her and said, "It is so helpful to talk with a professional about these matters." And he was sincere. Behind the mirror it seemed evident that the therapist was not responding to the couple but to her own ideas. This experience seemed to me to illustrate the possibility that a client would find deep meaning in random comments and interpretations of a therapist.

Supervisors should tolerate deviants in a training group but not if they behave in such extreme ways that their behavior is simply unacceptable. The supervisors should especially keep in mind the idea that the deviant trainee often expresses ideas the other group members are thinking but simply not saying. He or she is the spokesman for the unspoken objections of the group.

What About the *I Ching*?

One of the reasons for doing live supervision is to provide the supervisor with the opportunity to make use of his or her intuition. A supervisor gets

[2]Durkheim, E. (1951). *Suicide*. New York: Free Press.

ideas when seeing the composition of the therapist and the clients in the therapy room. When talking about a case with a trainee, a supervisor doesn't get an idea or an inner impulse in the same way. Could this be illustrated with the use of the *I Ching*?

Let me quote Allen Watts[3]:

> Traditional Chinese philosophy ascribes both Taoism and Confucianism to a still earlier source, to a work which lies at the very foundation of Chinese thought and culture, dating anywhere from 3,000 to 1,200 B.C. This is the *I Ching* of *Book of Changes*. It consists of oracles based on the various ways in which a tortoise shell will crack when heated. This refers to an ancient method of divination in which the soothsayer bored a hole in the back of a tortoise shell, heated it, and then foretold the future from the cracks in the shell so formed, much as palmists use the lines on the hand. For many centuries now the tortoise shell has fallen into disuse, and instead the hexagram appropriate to the moment in which a question is asked of the oracle is determined by the random division of a set of fifty yarrow stalks. But an expert in the *I Ching* need not necessarily use tortoise shells or yarrow stalks. He can "see" a hexagram in anything—in the chance arrangement of a bowl of flowers, in objects scattered upon a table, in the natural markings on a pebble. By far the greater part of our important decisions depend upon "hunch"—in other words upon the "peripheral vision" of the mind. Thus the reliability of our decisions rests ultimately upon our ability to "feel" the situation, upon the degree to which the "peripheral vision" has been developed. (pp. 13–15)

When a supervisor can actually see how a family is distributed in a room with the therapist, it's not unlike casting the yarrow stalks and observing the patterns they make. The answers aren't in the yarrow stalk patterns but in our minds as focused by the yarrow stalk or the sequences in client families. If a supervisor needs an idea, he or she can telephone the therapist and ask the therapist to move the family members to different chairs, such as moving the son out from between two parents. When that is done, the supervisor suddenly has an intuitive idea of what should be done with this family, just as if he had cast the stalks and observed the patterns.

It should be emphasized that supervisors should follow their impulses. An idea may come when a supervisor watches through the one-way mirror, and it should be acted on, even though at times the supervisor is in doubt about whether or not to follow that impulse. Later he or she may regret not doing so.

---

[3]Watts, A. (1957). *The way of Zen*. New York: Vintage Books.

Seeing the distribution of patterns through the mirror when looking at a family, like seeing the patterns when casting the *I Ching*, can be productive if one allows those patterns to focus one's intuition and if one acts on the impulse.

LIVE SUPERVISION EXAMPLE 1: BEING UNFAIR

A couple in their late 20s, who had been married about 7 years, came to therapy uncertain whether to stay together or separate. They were both dissatisfied, but neither one was willing to make a move to change their situation, particularly by moving toward the other. They were professional people and sophisticated about therapy.

The therapist was Ron Redman, a former minister with experience working with couples. Redman tended to bring out a couple's feelings about each other and offer straightforward advice. He was in training because he wished to learn the directive, brief approach to therapy. He presented himself in a professional manner with a somewhat folksy style. One of his primary characteristics was that he gave equal time to both spouses, having been taught that a therapist should be careful not to side with one spouse against the other.

In the first interview the problems and situation of the couple were explored. The wife said that her husband was dissatisfied and sulked. The husband said that his wife was ignoring him and that she was unhappy with the marriage. At home they often argued and shouted at each other. Although their families were involved with them, there appeared to be no in-law problems, and a decision about bringing in the parents was postponed. Both spouses were successful and devoted to their careers. The wife had recently taken a new position and was working long hours. When interviewed alone, she said she often stayed at work longer than was necessary because it was so unpleasant when she came home.

Spouses are seen individually as well as together in this approach, either in the first interview or at the beginning of the second. It is useful to have the information that each is unlikely to offer in the presence of the other spouse. For example, at times one spouse enters therapy with the wish to divorce and leave the other with the therapist rather than with a willingness to improve the marriage. Not knowing this can cause the therapist to waste time. There are issues of confidentiality when seeing spouses alone, but the advantages outweigh the disadvantages. A therapist should not be trapped into not revealing something, but generally there is nothing wrong with a therapist keeping secrets from one or both spouses and taking responsibility for what to do with those secrets.

There is another reason for seeing spouses separately: The therapist needs to be an authority to get things done, and authority requires power. One way to increase power is to control information. If a therapist only sees a couple in joint therapy sessions, both spouses know all that has been told to the therapist, but if the spouses are seen separately, neither knows what the other has said. But the therapist does. Since the therapist has more information than either spouse has, he or she has more power. When a couple is locked in a struggle, to get movement requires the therapist to have authority.

The focus of the presentation here is the second interview with the aforementioned couple. The first interview had ended without a directive, and the couple came back expecting further discussion of their dissatisfactions. The second interview began with such a discussion, with each spouse complaining to the therapist about the other. The discussion was the kind that sophisticated, articulate couples are able to carry on for many sessions if they are encouraged to do so, as often happens in private practice. In this directive, brief approach however, such articulate sophistication prevents change since change requires action.

When the husband said that he doubted his wife loved him, the therapist asked him for evidence of that. The husband said, "She absolutely avoids spending time with me, and she shows me very little warmth or affection, physically and emotionally." The wife interrupted and said, "That's not true." The husband insisted that it was, and continued, "I feel completely shut out of her life. I learn more about what's happening in her life by what I hear her telling people on the telephone. I don't feel that she wants to be around me at all. I think she is very close to moving out, wanting to be alone on her own, away from me." He added, "I've been trying real hard, and I don't get any positive feedback at all."

The therapist said, "How about when she reached out and touched you here? You didn't respond at all." The husband said, "I was aware of that. She wouldn't have done that at home." The wife interrupted angrily, "That's not true! It's an absolute lie!"

The therapist continued, "What evidence is there that she *does* love you?"

The husband replied, "Well, we're here, and we still live together."

The therapist asked, "Do you think she's interested in someone else?" (The wife, when seen alone, said that she was not.)

"I don't think that's the problem. No," said the husband.

The therapist said, "You feel you want more contact, and you're not getting it." "That's right," said the husband. "We're going through the motions, such as this therapy. Out of a sense of guilt or because the last step is a hard one to take."

"Letting you down softly?"

"Perhaps letting us both down softly. Feeling some responsibility to the marriage. At any rate, I don't feel very wanted."

Turning to the wife, the therapist said, "How about you? What is your view about whether he loves you or not."

"Oh, I think he loves me," she said. "I know he says he hates me every once in a while, but he tends to fly off the handle. Although it hurts me when he does that, certainly . . . a lot. I wish that he . . . the way I want somebody to show love is different from the ways which he tries to show it. And he's unwilling to show it in the ways I want it shown, because he doesn't feel that my ways are valid ways. I think we both have to come to terms with each other's way of showing it. And being able more readily to interpret how love comes across." She added, "I think he's losing patience with me. And I'm having a real hard time now."

"Do you think you'll have to go after him again? To court him again?"

"I don't know. Part of me doesn't want to. I feel like I shouldn't have to. If he's not willing to make a few changes here and there, I'm not going to be willing to do much either."

All couples have communication rules embedded in their relationship. What was becoming evident here was that the couple followed the rule that the wife is to initiate what happens, and the husband to respond. Sometimes relationship rules appear to be followed as inevitably as a train on a railroad track. For example, a couple can have a rule that the wife is responsible and the husband is irresponsible. Whatever they do, that rule is followed. If the wife wants to save money, the husband will want to spend it. If the wife wants to go to marriage therapy, the husband will avoid it (the sympathy of the therapist is usually with the wife because she says what a good client should say; whereas the husband won't even come in). And so on. Of course, the behavior of such a couple is mutually reinforcing in a systematic way: The more irresponsible the husband is the more responsible the wife becomes, and the more she is responsible the more irresponsible he becomes.

The rule followed by this couple that the wife is to initiate contact and the husband is to respond is a rule followed by many couples. Often, a couple is quite satisfied with that rule. However, if they become dissatisfied with it, a change becomes necessary. At a certain point in the marriage of this couple, the wife stopped initiating contact (as she said, "I feel I shouldn't have to") and began to wait for the husband to do so. He did not. The wife was then faced with the dilemma of having to decide whether to go back to initiating contact or to wait for her husband to do so, with the possibility that he might never come forward.

After about 20 minutes into the second interview, it became evident to the supervisor behind the mirror that nothing was happening in the therapy room except conversation. The couple was willing to talk forever about their ideas and feelings, but action needed to be taken for change to occur. The question was: Who should do what? The husband seemed to be waiting for the wife to initiate something; the wife, dissatisfied with being the initiator, was waiting for the husband to do something; both spouses were waiting for the therapist to do something, and the therapist was waiting for the supervisor to do something. Aware of the situation, the supervisor called the therapist out of the room for a consultation.

The supervisor understood that something had to be done to divert this therapeutic conversation into an action that would bring about change. Conversation does not change people unless there is a directive implicit in it. It seemed apparent to the supervisor that the couple wished to stay together, but that neither spouse was willing to take a step toward the other. The supervisor saw that that first step would need to be arranged by the therapist. The therapist, meanwhile, was actually preventing change by behaving in a neutral way, and so confirming the type of relationship the couple was revealing to him.

It is typical of married couples who come to therapy that one spouse has more power than the other. A primary way of determining who has power in a marriage is to note which spouse can threaten to leave the other. In this case, the wife could do so and apparently the husband could not. (Often one spouse will regularly threaten to leave the other over some issue, and the other will capitulate. However, if one day the one who regularly capitulate says, "All right. Let's separate," this upsets them both and they come for therapy.)

In this couple, the wife was in a superior position in relation to the husband. When she was dissatisfied, she went out and did things. The husband sat at home, frustrated, waiting for her. A therapist who is faced with this inequality and who behaves fairly and equally with both spouses is confirming their unequal relationship by being neutral. Neutrality indicates that no change is necessary, even though the therapist wishes this couple could change. Unfortunately, there is a tendency in marital therapy training to emphasize that the therapist should treat both spouses equally. The concern about inadvertently forming a coalition with one spouse against the other prevents the therapist from deliberately forming a coalition as part of the therapy. Yet by joining each spouse equally, when they are unequal with each other, the therapist is confirming their relationship instead of trying to change it.

It seemed obvious to the supervisor that this couple was locked in a systemic struggle in which each spouse's attempts to change the other only served to more tightly lock them in an unequal relationship. It also seemed apparent that the couple was prepared to talk about their relationship forever (or at least for many months). What was needed was some action that would destabilize them. The rigidity of their relationship suggested that the action would probably have to be extreme. To the supervisor the problem was not the couple but the therapist, who was committed to "fairness" and would have difficulty taking action if that action involved siding with one spouse against the other.

The group of trainees behind the one-way mirror seemed to think the interview was going well since the couple was expressing their feelings and articulating their differences. The structure of the situation, the inequality of the pair, their reluctance to take new actions—these were not obvious to them. Most of the trainees felt the therapist should continue the conversation, in which he was mainly encouraging the spouses to express their views. Their focus was on the couple, not on the triangle of couple and therapist. They were also unaware of the triangle involving the supervisor. Therefore, this was a good teaching situation.

A comment on thinking in terms of triangles is in order here. Some trainees have trouble learning to explain behavior in terms of triads, as any good therapist should. When a therapist sits down with a couple, the situation is a triangle. If a male therapist sees a wife in individual therapy, he is triangulating with the husband and wife in their marriage; the husband assumes his wife is talking to another man about him, which is so. When seeing a couple, the therapist has several choices. He or she can side with the wife against the husband, side with the husband against the wife, or try to be neutral. Each comment by a spouse pulls the therapist in that person's direction or drives the therapist away from a coalition with the person, and every comment to the couple by the therapist represents a coalition offered or declined. The birth of family-oriented marriage therapy began with the discovery that marriage therapy involves a triangle and that a couple changes when the therapist changes in relation to them. Before that discovery, marriage therapy focused on the couple as if the therapist were not there, which is a reflection of the belief that a marriage therapist must remain neutral (which is an impossibility in such a situation).

The therapist, like his supervisor, did not think the interview was going well. He was growing frustrated with the couple's repetitive complaints and was beginning to believe that something had to be done. He just didn't know what. His dissatisfaction made it possible for the supervisor to motivate him to change.

The Supervisor's Intervention

The supervisor said to the therapist, "Is it possible for you to be unfair?" The therapist wasn't sure what he meant. The supervisor clarified his question by asking him if he could choose one of the spouses and say that one was entirely wrong and the other was entirely right. The therapist replied that he didn't think he could do that, because it wasn't true. He said he believed that one spouse was never all wrong and the other all right, that spouses make misery conjointly. The supervisor agreed that that was probably true about the cause of marital misery but that it was not necessarily relevant to therapy. Understanding a cause does not necessarily lead to a hypothesis that is a guide to change.

At this point the supervisor told the therapist that he should side with one of the spouses against the other and tell them that one of them is wrong and the other right. However, this simple suggestion involved a series of stages before it was accepted, stages similar to those in which a therapist arranges an action with a client. The discussion between the therapist and supervisor was not recorded, but such an intervention typically involves a series of steps.

1. The supervisor talked with the therapist about how the couple was unhappy and he was obligated to help them change. He emphasized that, of course, the therapist wished to do this.
2. He suggested that if the therapy continues the way it was going, the couple would continue in their misery and not change.
3. He pointed out that the therapist had to do something because the couple was waiting for him to do something and that if he didn't have a plan, he would have to accept the supervisor's plan.
4. The supervisor said the plan to follow was to be unfair and say that one spouse is all wrong and the other all right.
5. He said the therapist had a good enough relationship with the couple that they would accept his intervention and not flee.

Part of the supervisor's agenda was to expand the range of the therapist. He was too predictable, which would be a problem with some clients. It took at least 10 minutes of discussion behind the mirror before the therapist agreed to be unfair. The supervisor gave him the choice of being unfair or failing with the case. A final comment seemed to help: The supervisor said that other therapists were able to be unfair. The therapist said that he could be as unfair as any other therapist, and he went into the interview room.

The question was: Which spouse should the therapist join against the other? Either one could be blamed for their troubled marriage, and ample evidence could be found to support any choice. The supervisor suggested that the husband be blamed. He should insist that the wife was not at fault at all and that the husband was the problem. This choice was made partly because the husband was not initiating in the relationship and could perhaps be persuaded to do so. This would please the wife, and her responses would ultimately please him. Another reason for choosing the husband was because of gender: It's easier for a male therapist to blame the husband and identify him as the problem. It can be done, of course, with a different gender arrangement, but this is the least complicated. When a female therapist blames the husband, this sometimes creates a situation where the husband feels ganged up on by two women. In that case the female therapist needs to partly escape gender by emphasizing her professional background; in that way the husband will not feel that he is being opposed by two women but by his wife and a professional. When properly trained, a therapist of either gender can choose among coalition approaches that deal satisfactorily with male–female issues.

The therapist and his supervisor planned the intervention before the clinical interview was resumed. He was to ask the couple to give therapy a chance for 3 months with no threat of separating during that period. Such a contract allows different changes to take place. Next, the therapist was to say to the husband that he was entirely wrong in the way he was dealing with the wife. He was to point out that she was not doing anything to create the problem and to insist that the husband save the marriage, which meant courting his wife to win her back because he was losing her.

Anticipating responses is part of this strategy. It was expected that the husband might say he didn't feel like courting his wife because things were so bad between them. Anticipating such a statement, the therapist was to tell the husband that he should at first pretend, if necessary, that he was in love with her, that he should go through the motions, if necessary, and that he would later develop the feelings. As the therapist discussed the therapy plan with his supervisor and understood more clearly what he was to do, he began to feel more enthusiasm. (Trainees are often reluctant to take a particular approach because they don't know how.) He returned to the therapy room committed to and capable of being unfair.

The Therapy Intervention

When the therapist told the couple that he would like to see them for a minimum of 3 months, the wife replied, half jokingly, "You mean that's all the time we get?"[4] From this remark the supervisor realized that there

---

[4]The dialogue presented here is verbatim, having been transcribed from the video recordings.

was another explanation for the couple's conversational approach to therapy. Often, a couple indicates by the way they introduce their problems that they plan long term therapy. That is, they talk in general ways about abstract issues. It is as if they are expecting to play a long game and see no reason to hurry and get to the point. By setting a period of time for the therapy the therapist can force a couple to deal with real issues in their lives.

The therapist replied to the wife that 3 months should be enough, and there was no rush since the problems had been going on for a while. Then the therapist said to the husband, "From what I heard tonight you really are in danger of losing your wife. I think what you are doing is absolutely wrong. I think you're making a mess of things. You are doing things to turn her off—by not talking to her, by not being aggressive, by not seeking her out, by not courting her." The husband sat still, looking solemn. The therapist added, "I think it's time you started courting her. You're driving her away to other systems, and to friends, letting her work those long hours, not spending time with her. You really need to . . . I would say, if I had to make a choice right now . . . I'd say you are absolutely wrong. It's your fault. If you want this woman as your wife, you have to get off your high horse and go after her and court her. You really have to take responsibility for this. And this is a good time of the year because it's spring and the sap is rising. I think this is the beginning of new life. This is the time to convince yourself, so that by 3 months you have it clear in your mind that you've done everything you can to win this woman as your wife. It's like a second marriage."

An observer would not know from the calm, firm, and kindly way the therapist delivered this intervention that it was difficult for him. Once he had decided the approach was necessary, he did it well and with enthusiasm. Looking at the wife, he added, "And it's no fault of yours." Turning to the husband, he said, "You might have to pretend in the beginning because you're still mad, still feeling cheated and ignored. You're going to have to pretend the first week or so that you are in love with her. Go through the motions. After you get into doing something, then you'll suddenly realize, 'Oh yeah, our marriage is getting better.' So I'm going to put the responsibility on you. You won't like what I'm saying—it's a hard message I'm giving you. And I don't see anything that your wife is doing that is contributing to this at all."

The wife interrupted, saying, "I must be doing something."

"No," said the therapist.

The husband sat forward and said, "Let's talk about this. I'm telling you, I think you're bullshit."

"No," insisted the therapist, "You really have to go after her and court her."

The husband said, with emotion, "She spends her time telling me that everything I am and everything I do is bad."

"You have to convince her that it's not," said the therapist. "You have to convince her by courting her, by meeting her at work, by calling her during the day."

"I call her during the day. I can't get through. She never returns calls. She's busy."

"Take time off and go meet her for lunch,"the therapist suggested. "Spend time with her, don't let her out of your sight. She's a prize possession. If this is the greatest thing in your life—it's better than margarine—then you better go after her because she's going to melt, she's going to disappear."

"That's right," said the husband, "I believe it."

"You really have to go after her . . . take the offensive here and go after her . . . and don't talk about criticism. She's just giving you a hard time."

"Yes, but her criticism is not just 'I don't like it when you do that,' but 'I'm going out.' "

"You go with her."

"I'm not invited."

"You don't have to wait for an invitation; you're the man of the house."

"She's not home. She comes home at 8:30 or 9:00 every night. I'm the first one home every night. What can I do? I'm there."

"Go to her office and meet her there."

At this point the supervisor phoned the therapist. While he was on the telephone, the wife reached out and stroked her husband's arm. (When a wife is absolved of all blame in her marriage, she has to come forward because she knows it's not true.) He responded by saying, "It's okay."

On the telephone the supervisor suggested that he not discuss abstractions with this husband but enumerate the specific things the husband could do the next day. As the therapist hung up the phone, the husband said, "That's a fairly bold statement after 2 hours," referring to the fact that his was only their second interview.

"I want you to think about this and pull out all the stops," said the therapist.

"We've thought about it," said the husband, referring to his wife and himself as a dyad.

"What will you do tomorrow to go after her so she doesn't slip through your fingers, so she's not moving away from you?" asked the therapist.

"Give up everything I believe in." said the husband.

"Well, you've got to modify that for the next 2 weeks."

"I probably won't do that."

"Well, what would prevent you . . . ? What could you do during the day tomorrow to convince her that she is the love of your life?"

"I'm not sure anymore."

"I realize it's hard for you at the beginning, because you're unsure."

"It's a certain type of person that she wants that I'm not. And I never will be."

"Can you be that for just tomorrow?"

"Well, what's the point? Because when I revert to myself, she'll go back to not liking me."

"Well, you can convince yourself that you can take on a new behavior. You're not locked in concrete. Because right now you guys are locked."

"That's right."

"One of you has got to change. By not changing, you're preventing her from responding to you. So you really have to take the first step and court her."

"I know what I have to do, and I've been doing it for the past few weeks. I have to show a lot of interest in her job but at the same time be very careful not to ask any questions that may be sensitive or suggest criticism or suggest that maybe she's not perfect. It's not allowed to have any kind of even-sided dialogue, but I'm supposed to be like I think her parents are. Just 'whatever you do is perfect.' And I'm not that kind of person."

"It would be hard for you. Then you'd have to pretend to be a good listener?"

"I'm not allowed to say, 'Well, what happened? What went on?' I'm just supposed to say, 'Oh, don't worry about it, you're wonderful, and what happened at work is bullshit,' and I'm not that kind of person."

"It strikes me that's not the type of person your wife is. It's being rude to her to say you can't get the facts out."

When a therapist unbalances this way, it is necessary to go to extremes. Not only is the wife absolved of blame, but if the husband criticizes her, the therapist should say that he is being rude and that the wife doesn't seem that way to him.

"I know everything about her job," said the husband. "I know the names of the employees, I know what's going on during the day, but I can't ask anything substantive. Something happens and the boss was upset and I'm not allowed. . . ."

The wife interrupted: "Because my boss yelled at me and I'm upset and the last thing I need is for my husband to turn around and examine me about the situation. I want you to say, 'It's okay.' "

"Just to be a listener, and not to give you the third degree. That would be hard for you," the therapist said to the husband.

"He could not do it," said the wife.

"It would be hard for me; it's not my personality."

"But you could learn that behavior, couldn't you?" asked the therapist.

The couple's dialogue changed with this intervention. They no longer talked in abstract intellectual terms. They began to straightforwardly negotiate change. The therapist continued to insist that the husband take action of a specific kind to court his wife, and his supervisor continued to phone in suggestions for different ways of telling the couple what should be done and for dealing with anticipated difficulties. For example, the therapist suggested that the husband might try to please his wife and then make a pass at her and she would reject him. But that would change if he continued to pursue her. This was done to avoid the situation where the husband might halfheartedly pursue this wife, then approach her sexually and have her reject him so that he would say the whole thing didn't work.

The husband then revealed that he had bought his wife a present the day before and was shopping that day for another. The therapist, keeping the pressure on the husband, replied, "Can you do more of that?" At one point in the interview the husband became quiet, and it seemed clear he was at the point of deciding whether to break up the marriage or take the actions he knew were necessary. One of the risks of this unbalancing approach is that it forces the issue of deciding the fate of the marriage. The husband was feeling that he and his wife could no longer just drift along, that he had to act, and that he had to decide if he was willing to take the steps necessary to save the marriage. At this point the wife, sensing the gravity of her husband's thoughts, became increasingly nervous. When she insisted that *she* ought to have to do something, the therapist replied that somewhere down the road something might be asked of her. Then he continued his relentless pursuit to change the husband, suggesting that he buy tickets and surprise his wife with a show, that he take her out to dinner, and so forth. When he wondered aloud if the husband might be angry at him, the husband shook his head. He knew the therapist was on his side and was only telling him what needed to be done. At one point the therapist asked the husband if he thought courting his wife would work to make a happier marriage. The husband replied, "I have no doubt about that." This statement obligated him to either make those efforts or leave the marriage. With encouragement, the husband came out of his silence and began to talk, apparently deciding the marriage was worth the effort.

As the interview ended, the therapist, at his supervisor's suggestion, asked the husband what color roses his wife liked. The husband replied that she didn't like roses. The wife coquettishly replied, "When did I ever say that?" The therapist suggested that her husband find out which flowers his wife liked.

At the next interview the couple came in cheerfully. Obviously there had been a change. The husband initiated the discussion of the week's events, and he described a number of his courting activities. (The therapist, at his supervisor's suggestion, had phoned the husband several times since the last interview to encourage him in his efforts to court his wife.) Both husband and wife had decided to take steps to change their marriage instead of being locked in a struggle in which neither was willing to make the first move.

LIVE SUPERVISION EXAMPLE 2: GETTING OUT OF A COALITION

A supervising problem occurred in the course of therapy with a young married couple.[5] The wife had become interested in another man and was uncertain whether to go with him or stay with her husband. The husband wanted his wife to remain with him, and although he was angry about the other man, he was trying to please and placate his wife.

The therapist was having difficulty helping the couple resolve this impasse. A supervising problem was that the therapist was siding with the wife against the husband. The therapist had begun by seeing the wife in an individual interview and saw her alone for a second hour because he was impressed with how complex and interesting her situation was. When the therapist brought in the husband, he saw the husband alone to balance the relationship with both spouses. The therapist was already quite sympathetic to and fond of the wife, and even seeing the husband alone did not change his attitude. Ostensibly, the therapist was being even-handed with the couple, but covertly he and the wife both felt that the husband wasn't quite up to what he should be. This coalition seemed to prevent the husband from taking action. For example, the husband said that he was trying to win his wife back by paying more attention to her. Now when his wife spoke to him, he would put down the newspaper and listen to her. When I, as the supervisor in this case, heard these words from behind the one-way mirror, I did not think that such behavior constituted a very powerful move on the part of the husband to win his

[5]The report of this case is adapted from Haley, J. (1988). Reflections on supervision. In H. A. Liddle, D. C. Breunlin, & R. C. Schwartz (Eds.), *Handbook of family therapy training and supervision* (pp. 358–367). New York: Guilford Press.

wife, particularly a wife who had been having an affair with a romantic
and attentive man.

There are at least three ways to view the minimal efforts of this
husband. One can assume that he was ignorant and didn't know how to
interest his wife in a romantic way (which therapy could teach him). Or
he might be angry at his wife for the affair. Or he might have been
responding to the social situation that includes the therapist; that is, he
might have been reluctant to make a dramatic move to win his wife when
she and the therapist seemed to be patronizing about his efforts. For
example, when the therapist asked the wife, in a kindly way, "Don't you
consider your husband to be making an effort to win you back?" she
replied reluctantly, "I guess." When a husband assumes a wife and
therapist are covertly against him, he will not extend himself to win back
the wife, particularly if that's what the therapist seems to want.

It seemed evident to me that the therapist had involuntarily triangulated on the side of the wife in such a way that change was being
prevented. The wife couldn't make up her mind whether to stay with her
husband or go with the other man. The husband was angry at the
therapist and his wife and only halfheartedly made efforts to save his
marriage. The therapist was under pressure from me to resolve the
problem and was hesitant to act because he didn't know what I wanted.
I hadn't come up with anything to help the therapist out. Everyone was
stuck.

A supervisor in such a case might discuss with the trainee the nature
of marriage, the issue of extramarital involvements, the stages of marriage, and so on, but with an emphasis on gathering more information.
The question of how to change this couple would be avoided in such
reflective discussions. A supervisor focused on the personality of the
therapist would point out to him that he was siding with the wife against
the husband and might suggest personal therapy. Perhaps such a supervisor would offer to examine with the therapist his own marriage, on the
assumption that the therapist's own marital difficulties were creating a
problem for him in his clinical work. Perhaps the supervisor would have
the trainee simulate his own marriage, or even his parent's marriage, in
an effort to help him work through his dilemma in dealing with this
couple.

A supervisor might also assume that this sort of situation often
happens and that any therapist might at some time get into an involuntary coalition with one spouse against the other. This is one of the
consequences of doing marital therapy, and even prominent therapists
can find themselves in such a coalition.

The supervisor's task is to disengage therapists from an unhelpful
coalition if they cannot do it themselves. Whether the therapist's own

marriage was troubled would not be considered relevant or allowed as an excuse. Emotional problems shouldn't interfere with a therapist's work. Moreover, a supervisor would also assume that therapists do not need insight into the fact that they are in coalition with a client against a client's spouse. The therapist already knows that. The problem is doing something about it. If the coalition is insightfully presented by the supervisor as his or her problem, it could cause harm. To please the supervisor, such a therapist is likely to withdraw from the wife and try to side with the husband. The "abandoned" client would then wonder what he or she had done wrong, and the newly joined spouse would sense that what the therapist was offering was artificial and phony.

Behind the one-way mirror with a group of trainees, I watched the therapist and the wife rather patronizingly talk to the husband about how he was trying to please his wife but wasn't quite up to it. I was looking for some way to change the balance of the couple in relation to the therapist. The husband was in a weak position while the wife was in a strong position, because of the therapist's support of her. The therapist needed to put the wife down and lift the husband up by changing his relationship with them. But he had to do it in a way that didn't offend or reject the wife. I was assuming that the couple couldn't change in relation to each other until the therapist changed in relation to them, and that the therapist was not likely to change in relation to them until I changed in relation to him.

As I searched for a directive, a female in the group of trainees behind the mirror with me mentioned that the wife was presenting herself as not very feminine. Indeed, she was wearing a man's work shirt and jeans. "Perhaps," said the trainee, "she is dressing that way to keep her husband at a distance." I found that observation helpful and telephoned the therapist. I suggested that he say to the husband that he would know when he was successful in pleasing his wife when she responded to him in a more feminine way.

The therapist repeated that remark to the couple, and the wife immediately said she did not agree with it. Coming to life for the first time in the interview, the husband looked pleased and said he appreciated the comment. The wife protested that if her husband wanted a more feminine woman, he would have to look elsewhere. The therapist said he just thought he'd mention this point, and he went on to other matters.

After that simple intervention, the wife and husband behaved toward each other as equals, and the therapist was no longer in coalition with the wife. At the next interview the husband insisted that his wife make her choice of him or the other man. He apparently saved that ultimatum to be given in the presence of the therapist, whom he now trusted to be fair. The wife made her choice.

A particular supervision question is raised by this example. The therapist followed the directive of the supervisor and found himself free of the handicapping coalition, but he didn't understand what had happened. In this therapy approach clients are not usually told why or how an intervention leads to change. Should the supervisor tell the trainee? Is nonawareness therapy logically taught by nonawareness training? Many therapists are now comfortable with the idea that they can change a family without the family's awareness of how the change came about. It might logically follow that a supervisor may change the problem of a trainee by manipulating him or her outside awareness.

The goal of a therapist is to resolve family problems. Awareness of how a therapist accomplishes this need not be shared with the family if such awareness might interfere with the change. In the present case the therapist might inform the couple that he made the remark about feminine appearance to support the husband in a more equal relationship with the wife. Although their response is not predictable, as one wishes responses to be, the odds are such a comment would antagonize both of them. This antagonism would interfere with the next steps in the therapy. Therapists who try to be totally honest with a client typically end up as not respected. The therapy context is not like other situations where honesty is appropriate, as among friends.

The question of whether or not awareness should be offered to a trainee therapist can be determined by the goals of the therapists and the supervisor. Should I, as the supervisor in this case, have explained to the therapist why he became disengaged from the coalition with the wife if he didn't know? Although the machinery of the therapy is not the domain of the client, it is of the therapist. My task as supervisor was not only to help the trainee change this couple but also to teach him how to change troubled couples in the future. To achieve that goal, some conceptualization of his involvement with the family was necessary. However, one should note that many expert therapists are not conceptualizers. As a professional therapist watcher, I have gone over recordings of therapy sessions with many competent therapists. I have learned that a therapist knows what to do in a case but may have difficulty offering reasons when he or she is asked to explain the rationale for a particular intervention. It would be ideal if therapists developed a theory of therapy and then carried therapy out in a series of steps demanded by the theory. It seems, however, more often it happens that therapists take actions in therapy and later design a theory to explain the success of their actions. Many who teach therapists use metaphors, such as case examples, to describe a situation that is too complex for a digital explanation.

Therapists who are willing to accept the idea that therapy is a process of influence and therefore a process of manipulation must decide if supervision can be thought of in the same way. If one changes clients outside their awareness, is it acceptable to train therapists in the same way? Everyone must take a position. One way to think about the matter is this: What happens in the therapy room can be so complex that conscious conceptualization as one works is improbable.

In the case example presented here I explained to the therapist why I had suggested that he make the comment about the wife responding in a more feminine way and why I thought it helped him disengage from his coalition with her. He corrected the imbalance without offending the wife, and the husband became more equal to her in terms of a relationship to the therapist. I'm not sure that this explanation was necessary for the therapist to solve a similar situation in the future. The action itself could have been sufficient.

It would seem to be best for supervisors to have the freedom to influence trainees outside their awareness, particularly if making them aware of an intervention would oversimplify it or interfere with their learning it. It is different if the trainee is to become a teacher or supervisor. In that case he or she must learn the conceptualizations in order to pass them on. Thus, the process of learning how to teach is itself a learning situation.

The principle is the same as when conducting therapy. The difference is that a trainee therapist must learn to influence many kinds of people in many situations and thus needs education as a people changer. The family just needs to know how to live together without a special problem.

LIVE SUPERVISION EXAMPLE 3:
HOW TO APOLOGIZE TO YOUR PATIENT
FOR CAUSING HIM IRREVERSIBLE
BRAIN DAMAGE

When communication was discovered in the interpersonal era, it began to be taken for granted that what a patient said was in response to what the therapist said or did, even though at times the connection was obscure. If a patient said, "The refueling ship was late in meeting my submarine this morning," it was assumed that this was a comment on the therapist being late. It seemed evident that patients often felt that the safest way to communicate is in metaphor, since one cannot then be accused of criticizing, which may happen when comments are stated directly. With the arrival of the mind altering drugs in the 1960s, psychiatry once again began to accept a patient's statements as mere expressions of disordered thinking and not as responses to the social situation. This was a great relief to those therapists who didn't like what patients were implying with their metaphors. Strange communication from a patient was again received as only an indication to the psychiatrist that a drug was necessary in the treatment and regimen. The only question that remained was: Which drug will best stop this way of talking and get this person under social control? Psychiatric communication began to be pharmacological.

At times, the fact that a client's odd statements are a comment on the therapist simply cannot be ignored, no matter how much the therapist might prefer to do so. A therapist may try to deny that the client is speaking in metaphor or is expressing a criticism in courtesy language, but there are still instances when he or she simply cannot pretend that the client's remarks are only an expression of a thought disorder. When the client repeatedly pursues the therapist with the same metaphor, important ideas are being communicated. Sometimes the client and therapist can be locked in a game of avoiding the unfortunate issues implied in the psychotic language. Therapy then becomes interminable unless a supervisor steps in and saves them both from their impasse.

Reginald was a plump man in his 20s, who exasperated everyone by insisting that he had committed a murder. He particularly exasperated his therapist, Dr. X, a psychiatric resident, because he talked about little else besides the murder during three years of individual therapy. Dr. X patiently listened to Reginald explain again and again and again that he had killed someone and was being followed, usually by men in a black car who were, he suspected, FBI agents. When asked for details about the murder, Reginald was a little vague, claiming amnesia for much of what happened, but he was certain that he was a murderer and ultimately would be punished for it, and that the men in the black car would move in and take him away.

Reginald had been hospitalized several times over the years. During much of his adulthood, he'd been medicated with powerful antipsychotic drugs. As a result of the medication, he had tardive dyskinesia, a form of neurological damage brought on by neuroleptics. His symptoms were typical of this psychiatric disorder and included involuntary movement of the lips and hands and an involuntary flicking of the tongue. If Reginald concentrated on stopping the movement of his hands, he could do so, but when his thoughts went elsewhere the movement began again. His lip movements gave his face an ugly grimace. Except for the dyskinesia and his fear of the fellows in the black car coming to get him for murder, his other problem was that he wouldn't go to work to support himself.

Entering a family therapy training program, Dr. X brought Reginald for live supervision. The supervisor had Dr. X see Reginald together with his family. The father was a physical invalid with diabetes and the mother was not well. It seemed evident that one of the reasons Reginald did not work to support himself was because he was staying at home to take care of his father. In addition to physical care, he also provided his father with something to think about so that he wouldn't be depressed about his illness. Indeed, Reginald's father often expressed exasperation about this supposed murder in rather colorful language, and his anger helped him forget that his illness was incurable and would probably lead to the loss of his legs. In family sessions the father said he didn't need Reginald at home taking care of him. The mother agreed that she could care for her husband herself. Reginald enrolled in a job rehabilitation program, and he began to be away from home during the day, like any working person. His parents survived well without him. However, Reginald continued to talk to both his parents and the therapist about the murder and those fellows in the black car. The father and mother told the therapist that Reginald was driving them out of their minds by his talk of this crime.

At the supervisor's suggestion, the therapist persuaded the parents that they no longer needed to be tolerant, for the sake of their sick son, of Reginald's incessant monologue about the supposed murder. At the therapist's insistence, the parents agreed in a family session that if Reginald told them one more time about this murder, they would immediately call a lawyer and present the case to him. That is, they would treat the murder as a real event for which legal defense was necessary. (Often taking a metaphor literally is helpful to these cases.) The parents persisted in this plan, even when Reginald protested that the lawyer would be expensive and would probably ridicule them. The parents not only agreed to the plan, but were enthusiastic about it. It was the first time they had received practical advice about what to do to stop Reginald's repeated discussion of the murder.

Only once did Reginald mention the murder to his parents after this family therapy session. They immediately began to call a lawyer. Reginald argued with them, since he did not want them to spend the money, and promised not to mention the crime to them again—and he didn't. Apparently he received his parents determination to stop such talk as an indication that they didn't need that form of "assistance" from him. This response illustrates how normal a psychotic young person can become when his parents agree with each other and refuse to tolerate certain behaviors. However, in individual therapy sessions Reginald continued to exasperate his therapist with repetitive talk about the murder.

With the help of his supervisor, Dr. X made a plan for dealing with Reginald's crime. Reginald had said that it was fortunate that he was crazy. If he were normal, the men in the black car would come and get him and put him on trial for murder. The therapist was advised to take this seriously and to talk to Reginald about what a problem this was for him, the therapist. Often it is helpful for therapists to take metaphors personally.

As an aside, let me describe another case in which it was quite helpful to take a metaphor literally. I was doing therapy in a Veterans Administration hospital with a patient who had been diagnosed as chronic schizophrenic and who had been locked up for a number of years. I was seeing him an hour a day, which is how some inpatient therapists worked in the 1950s. We thought long-term therapy meant deep therapy. This patient—we'll call him Sam—was a "word salad" young man; that is, he talked at great length in what seemed to be random metaphors. I made interpretations to him, without any particular effect. One exasperating problem was Sam's insistence that he was rich and had millions of dollars put away. In fact, he was a migratory laborer who had gone mad and had been put in a state hospital. Later he was transferred to a VA hospital when he gave an army serial number that happened to be accurate, unlike other facts about himself, such as his birthplace, which he said was Mars.

Sam's discussion of being rich and having millions intruded into our therapeutic dialogues, and I was becoming more and more exasperated with this topic. Finally, I decide to take action. I had begun to invite Sam to my home for dinner to give him some experience outside hospitals, for he had been locked up for so many years that he didn't remember how to live on the outside. My children enjoyed him and appreciated his wild metaphoric discussions, taking them to be interesting stories. During a therapy session after one such visit, when Sam began his discussion of being a millionaire, I said that since he had visited my home, he could see that I wasn't a wealthy person, and since he had so much money, I thought it would be nice if he gave me a million dollars to pay off my mortgage. I said, "Why don't you come in this Friday with a million?" Friday he came in with a roll of Monopoly money. I pointed out that this wasn't really money, and it wouldn't be accepted for my mortgage payment. I said I was disappointed in him for not helping me with my personal finances. I thumbtacked the bill to the wall of my office. Only once after that did Sam mention being rich. I merely pointed to the bill on my wall, and he never mentioned being rich again. The whole metaphor was gone, and we began to make plans for him to leave the hospital and find work.

I told the psychiatric resident, Dr. X, that he should take Reginald's metaphor about murder literally. And he did so by asking Reginald what would happen to him if he was helped to become normal, Reginald said he would probably go to jail for murder. The therapist replied that that made the therapy impossible, since he, as a therapist, had the goal of helping Reginald get back to normal. "You'll get a job," Dr. X told him, "you'll do real well for a year or so, and then you'll be sent off to jail." Dr. X told Reginald that he didn't want all the work of helping him become normal only to have him go to jail on a murder charge. "Maybe what you should do instead of going through all that is to turn yourself in to the police right now," said Dr. X. "Serve your time and then get a job. If the arrest is really going to happen, maybe that's what you should do."

Reginald considered the matter thoughtfully, leaning forward with his elbows on his knees and holding his hands together as he always did, so they wouldn't tremble. "Well, I have a lead on a job," he said, "and I'm going to get it if I can." He explained that vocational rehabilitation was offering him a job. "I'm not going to turn myself in," he said. "If they want me, they can come and get me. They know where I'm at. If they don't want me, they'll leave me alone. I don't give a damn one way or the other."

The therapist persisted, "Well, I suggest you turn yourself in. Get it over with. It would be tough for me to see you go to jail just when you're doing well. Like you said, you'll get a job and start advancing at it, and then bang—you're off to jail."

"You think that will really happen?" asked Reginald.

"You said so yourself. If you're normal, that is going to happen."

Reginald became thoughtful and said again that he didn't want to go to jail just when he was about to get a job. Dr. X repeated his recommendation. "You're normal in many ways," he said, "But you still have those thoughts about the murder. Let's agree that if those thoughts bother you again, you'll just go turn yourself in and get it off your mind."

"Okay," said Reginald doubtfully.

The supervisor, observing from behind the mirror became increasingly puzzled about why Reginald continued to exasperate his therapist with this delusion about having murdered someone. The family situation had improved to the point where the young man didn't seem to need to be crazy, he was learning a trade, and he had a serious job offer. He was making a few friends, and was even exercising to get himself in better physical shape. Yet he continued with his repetitive talk of the murder and the men in the black car. It was also puzzling why Dr. X seemed so tolerant as he listened patiently to this repeated talk of murder, despite his boredom with it. For years, hour after hour, he had listened to these stereotyped phrases. Of course, the supervisor was assuming this wasn't just an expression of thought disorder but a communication with meaning, a mystery.

The supervisor called Dr. X out of the room to discuss the puzzle of why the young man persisted with his talk of murder. The therapist was also puzzled. "Tell me," said the supervisor, "who was treating Reginald when he got tardive dyskinesia?" "I was," said Dr. X. "I was treating him as part of an experimental drug program, and he developed the dyskinesia. That's why I've been doing therapy with him the last three years . . . because I felt so guilty about that."

The supervisor had discovered a clue to the mystery. It was reminiscent of other situations where a patient and doctor become locked in a struggle they can't resolve. A typical situation: A patient is treated for pain and becomes addicted to the pain medication. The doctor, in exasperation and guilt over the addiction, attempts to cut the patient off from the medication at the point where there is no longer a physical cause for the pain. Angry with the doctor because of the addiction, the patient continues to have the pain. Sometimes such patients will go from doctor to doctor in their community getting pain medication for this hysterical pain and letting the medical community know that their doctor didn't cure them, but instead addicted them to a drug.

The supervisor talked to Dr. X about his ethical responsibility to apologize to Reginald for having harmed him with medication. It seemed possible that Reginald was paying him back for causing his tardive dyskinesia, and the way he was paying him back was by not allowing him to cure the delusion about murder. The solution seemed obvious. "You're going to have to go in and apologize to him," the supervisor said. "Are you up to it?"

The therapist agreed to apologize to the young man for the damage he had done to him three years before. He returned to the therapy room but had difficulty doing this task. He talked to Reginald about how well he was doing, and then he said, "You know, sometimes with people with similar problems we do different types of therapy. One thing we use is medicine . . . medication."

"Yeah," said Reginald.

"And we've talked before about the side effect you have."

"Yeah."

After a long pause, Dr. X said, "You know, you're doing fine, and yet you have this tardive dyskinesia. It's a tough thing to have."

"Yeah."

"I've been seeing you off and on for several years. The first time I saw you, when you were hospitalized, we used Haldol."

"Yeah."

"And that seemed to work pretty well that first time."

"Uh-huh."

"The second time you came in the hospital, I was involved in your treatment again. We used that new drug."

"Mmmm."

"You had a lot of side effects with that, as I recall. Pacing up and down, that kind of stuff."

"I don't remember," said the young man.

"Yeah, well I do," said the therapist sadly. "I do."

"Okay."

"You know, for a doctor to . . . sometimes we think that what we do is good for a patient, and it turns out not to be." With a sigh, the therapist continued: "The problem is, I feel terrible. I feel terrible about you. About you having this side effect."

"I don't notice that I have the side effect, really," said the young man softly.

"The movements of your fingers and the lip movements. When you think about it you can control it, but when you're busy with something else you've probably noticed that your fingers will move and you have those lip movements. Personally, I feel terrible about that."

"Why should you feel terrible?"

"Well, you know, I gave you something that I thought was going to help."

"It did at the time."

"Yes, but then it had this side effect." After a pause, Dr. X said, "The thing is, it happened to *you*."

"Yeah," said Reginald sadly, "That it did. It did happen to me."

"What do you think about it?"

After a pause, Reginald said, "There's not much that can be done. You can't change anything. Everything has already been done. Unfortunately, God just can't do it. Some things are irreversible, I guess you might say."

"Yes," said the therapist, "at this point there's no way to reverse it. And I don't know—one can't predict the future."

Reginald changed the subject. He had been talking earlier about the difficulty his parents were having coming to the hospital for the interviews because of their physical infirmities. Now he said he thought his parents didn't need to continue to come regularly. Reginald said, "Suppose we meet only one more time with my mother, all three of us here, and that will be the end of the family sessions. I think I'm going to stop seeing you myself, if that's okay with you." After a pause, he continued, "Because really, I think you've done all you can really do for me. I don't think you can do any more. You've helped me back to the point where I can function."

The therapist faced a dilemma. He knew, of course, that it's always good if a patient is willing to become independent and no longer needs therapy, but he was uncertain of the motive behind Reginald's desire to end his therapy at this time. Dr. X was concerned that Reginald's decision meant that the young man felt it was hopeless to try to achieve any more and that he was asking him to corroborate this conclusion. The supervisor then telephoned in some advice, and Dr. X said to Reginald, "I can't let you go that easily. I can't let your family go that easily. The fact is, you're doing so well now, but I don't want to stop until I see you completely back to normal."

"Yeah," said Reginald,"I think I'm doing wonderful. I feel pretty good. I don't have murderous thoughts that often. Once in a while, once in a great while. I try not to let it bother me. I try to do something else, you know."

These words were said to the therapist as a kind of present, indicating to him that his patient's troublesome thoughts were going away, and that he was perhaps expressing appreciation for his therapist's apology. Dr. X said, "I think we should meet with your folks occasionally and you should go ahead with the job program."

Dr. X then discussed a proposed schedule of exercise and social life for Reginald. Toward the end of the interview he returned to the earlier topic: "If those thoughts start to bother you, you turn yourself in. Free your mind of that. Are you clear on that."

"If I have thoughts like that, I just pick up and turn myself in?" asked Reginald.

"If it's going to hassle you, yeah. The thing is, you're normal now, and that's the important thing."

Reginald said, "I don't think I murdered anyone; only crazy people do that. It's insane." He gave a little laugh.

"Okay," said the therapist.

"You're not going to release me from the therapy yet?"

"Not until you're out making a living. I'm not giving up."

Reginald smiled. "I really appreciate your help," he said—a surprising statement from this young man.

Reginald got a job and became self-supporting. Dr. X continued to see him and to see the young man's parents, often stopping at their house on the way home from the hospital in the evening since they could only get about with difficulty. The fellows in the black car disappeared.

9

SIMILARITIES BETWEEN THERAPY AND SUPERVISION

It is possible to consider the techniques of therapy and the techniques of supervision as synonymous. All the innovative therapy interventions being developed today to help clients can be used to help trainee therapists. Once one accepts the idea that therapy should be directive, the directives become available, for trainees as well as for clients.

Since the social context induces ideas and emotions in the clients, it follows that the social context can be a source of problems with trainees. Suppose a trainee is having difficulty accepting and acting on a supervisor's ideas. Today we would approach the problem by investigating whether the trainee is caught between two supervisors who are in conflict. We would also consider the possibility of a conflict between the ideas of the trainees personal therapist and those of a supervisor who has new ways of thinking about therapy. Being inadequate is a way for the trainee to satisfy these conflicting relationships. That is, the trainee is like the problem person in family therapy who is caught between authorities in the family and becomes inadequate.

In the past a person trained in the view of traditional therapy would explain the problems of client and the problems of therapists in terms of the theory of repression. A difficulty with that framework is its negative view of people. A therapist should have a positive view to offer clients. What people can do is more important than what they cannot do. Many trainees go through personal therapy, for which they are required to remember everything that was awful in their lives and conclude that this experience must be a good thing to impose on their clients, particularly if they are encouraged in this by a supervisor. Today supervisors must oppose such a conclusion. (Trainees with a traditional background also hesitate to make plans with a client for a therapy session or even for the therapy itself. They were taught to wait and see what the client does, that is, to be spontaneous reactors instead of planners.)

Therapists who use brief, directive therapy make plans, use directives, and assume that conversation does not change symptoms, that action must be taken. If a trainee has difficulty with a client, talking about it with a supervisor usually will not resolve the difficulty unless there is an implicit directive from the supervisor in the conversation. Discussing ideas and ideology leads to more discussion of ideas and ideology. Some supervisors like to discuss the meaning of a trainee's problems with the trainee and can become exasperated when the discussion does not resolve them; they may even scold the trainee, although they would never do this to a client. There are still supervisors who are unwilling to tell a trainee what to do (these supervisors were taught to avoid being directive with clients); they think of a trainee who gets stuck as one who has emotional problems rather than as one who lacks skill or is responding to an inhibiting social context.

In the past many supervisors knew how to be philosophical but didn't know how to teach trainees to be effective. Now we are in an era when the supervisor must know what to do—or make a brave try. The therapy approach taught and the procedures followed in a training program should be consistent. When therapy involved insight and focused on the unconscious, supervision did also. Now that therapy is becoming brief and active and uses a variety of directives the approach used in training has similar characteristics. The problems of the trainee are resolved by changes in relation to the supervisor, just as the client's problems are resolved in relation to the therapist. The techniques of brief therapy are available to the therapy teacher. Supervisors can use problem-solving orientation or a solution emphasis; they can restrain trainees from changing as a way to change them, or make use of paradox or metaphors, or offer an ordeal, or use straightforward advice and directives. Supervisors can be as active and directive as therapists are now expected to be. They can use straightforward directives with trainees, such as advice and coaching, and if a trainee has a problem and "can't help it," supervisors can use indirect techniques, just as they would with a client who "can't help it."

THE USE OF PARADOX

The following personal example illustrates the use of paradox: In a live supervision program I supervised a young therapist who was so nervous that it was interfering with the therapy she was doing with a family. She was constantly afraid of making mistakes and overconcerned with my opinion of her. Her nervousness was apparent not only to me but to the family. There was a danger that her anxiety would cause her clients to lose respect for her. She behaved as if she couldn't help herself. Something had to be done.

If a supervisor made interpretations to her about the personal reasons behind her anxiety, she might feel even less adequate. Moreover, a recommendation that she have personal therapy to recover from her problem would not have helped the particular family she was interviewing and would have been a cop-out by me. Helping her carefully prepare her interviews didn't seem to make her less nervous. Assuring her that she was doing a competent interview, which was so, didn't allay her anxiety in the therapy room. She continued to express her fear of making a mistake, like bringing up the wrong subject or offering a solution too soon or joining the child against the mother, and so on.

It was apparent that coaching and straightforward directives weren't solving this problem. I decided to use an indirect technique, as one might with a client. Just before a therapy interview I said to her, "You are worried about making mistakes. I want to help you get over that worry. Today when you go into the room with the family, I want you to make three mistakes." The young woman, startled, said, "Three mistakes?" "Yes," I said. "These must be special mistakes. I want one of the mistakes to be one that you and I both know is a mistake." "Okay," she said, taking notes. "I want you to make that mistake correctly," I said. "The second mistake is to be one that I wouldn't know is a mistake, but that you know is a mistake. It will be your personal mistake. Finally I want you to make a mistake that you don't know is a mistake." I added firmly, "I want you to make all these mistakes correctly." "All right," she said nervously, writing down these instructions as the family entered the interview room behind the mirror. The young woman conducted a reasonably competent interview, but she seemed thoughtful and preoccupied. When she came out after the interview I asked firmly, "Did you make all those mistakes correctly?" "Fuck you," said the young woman—and she was not so nervous in the future.

Therapists inexperienced with the effective use of paradox might wonder why the trainee didn't protest that she couldn't make a mistake she herself didn't know was a mistake, or why she didn't protest that I was using paradox with her. It should be recognized that a paradox is effective at a relationship level. A trainee who is having an exaggerated response to a supervisor is not likely to criticize the supervisor's words. My trainee couldn't argue that it was impossible for her to make a mistake she didn't know was a mistake. That would have meant correcting me, and she couldn't do that because of her fears. If she had questioned how she could make such a mistake, I would have told her she had to figure it out for herself or perhaps I would have explained that she could make a mistake without realizing it. If she had accused me of using paradox on her—which she wouldn't do—I would have agreed with her and would have told her to follow my directions carefully in order to fully understand that.

There are two aspects to the use of paradox that are important: One uses a paradox on those with whom it will be effective (the paradox used with this young woman might not be used with another trainee). The other major point is that awareness that a paradox is being used does not make it ineffective with the subject. Sometimes a client will say, "You're using reverse psychology on me." The proper reply is, "Yes, that's one of the things I'm doing." When I was in practice my colleagues would sometimes say, "I have this symptom; would you do a paradox on me?" If they did what I said, the paradox was effective; this is because paradox works at a relationship level, not an awareness level.

Supervisors lacked skill in giving directives to trainees because they themselves were trained in the nondirective age. For example, a trainee might have difficulty dealing with older women; he or she might have trouble being authoritative with them. The same trainee might not have that problem with younger women. The supervisor can't merely wish the trainee would get over the difficulty or even recommend that the trainee go into personal therapy to resolve problems with his or her mother. It's the supervisor's job to teach the trainee how to deal effectively with women and men of any age. For years insight-oriented supervisors blamed trainees' emotional problems rather than their lack of training for such difficulties. That was a way of avoiding having to teach what to do.

A range of possible directives used in therapy is available to the supervisor for training. The goal is to change the behavior of the therapist so that he or she can make use of a broad range of interview skills. Just as the therapist formulates a client's problem and intervenes, so too does the supervisor focus on formulating the trainees' technical problems and intervene to change them.

STAGES OF TRAINING

As with therapy, training occurs in stages and should be built on a positive relationship. The stages of training include the following:

1. The supervisor behaves in a nonthreatening way to help the trainees feel at ease.
2. The supervisor should offer a contract stating that basic ideas

will be taught and the trainees will learn a new approach to therapy.

3. Trainees are taught beginning directives to organize a family or bring out an individual.
4. The trainees are observed in action and the supervisor will formulate their problems in conducting a therapeutic interview.
5. Interventions are made to improve the trainees.
6. Trainees' development is followed to avoid relapse to behaviors learned prior to this training.

Trainees range from beginners just starting to do therapy to experienced therapists who wish to learn a particular therapy approach. Each trainee is a unique teaching problem, but a few generalizations can be made. Beginners face a dilemma: They wish to look like they know what they're doing, but they have to concede that there's a lot they don't know in order to learn. Experienced therapists have the same dilemma in a more extreme form: They don't want to be treated as novices, but inasmuch as they are learning a new approach, they *are* novices. They are tempted to show off their knowledge but much of that knowledge is incorrect in this new approach and their views are likely to be corrected. For example, experienced therapists might be more comfortable conducting individual interviews because of their lack of experience with family interviews. Therefore they find an ideological excuse for seeing family members alone, even when it's not appropriate. The supervisor needs to change this by helping trainees gain confidence in their interview skills with families. Then their ideas, too, will change. The supervisor needs to demonstrate in the training the same ideas being taught in the therapy: People's ideas change when their social situation changes.

BEGINNING THE TRAINING

Supervisor's must show concern and understanding that gives trainees enough support so they are able to follow directives and risk trying innovations. When trainees arrive in a group, they should be made comfortable and offered hope that the training will be an interesting and valuable experience. It helps if they have a room that is their own territory during the training period. (If a female trainee carries her purse into a therapy room, one can infer that she does not believe her place is her own behind the one-way mirror.) Trainees should also feel that the interview room itself is their territory. Sometimes permitting trainees to practice an opening speech—such as introducing the one-way mirror and the cameras to a family—in the therapy room gives the trainee the feeling that that room is their domain (as well as the experience of making an efficient opening with a client). While it is common for clients to feel as if they are in someone else's territory when they enter the therapy room, trainees shouldn't feel that way.

There are a variety of possible schedules for training. One of the most effective for working therapists is to train them all day one day a week. They can observe many families in the course of an entire day and thus be exposed to a great variety of clinical problems over the year. If families are scheduled for an hour and a half, it is possible in this span of time to plan the interview, have an hour's interview, and then have a discussion with the therapist afterward.

It is best to supervise every interview of a trainee. There are training programs where the trainee is supervised on the first interview but not again for several interviews (or perhaps never again with the same family). The difficulty with this arrangement is that the trainee lacks supervision for each stage of the therapy. Moreover, if the therapist gives the client a directive, the supervisor who observes the trainee once cannot know how it was carried out or how the trainee reacted. Supervision for every interview is the most expensive kind of training, but the intensity of such a program pays off. The trainee is guided through the initiation of change in a client and reaction to that change, which is the crucial period of therapy.

When a trainee is employed and receives training one day each week, he or she can take what is learned each day and apply it the next day on the job. In contrast, trainees who are not working therapists cannot immediately put into practice what they are learning. Often agencies will allow employees one day off per week for training—and even pay for it—particularly if they see results.

When the group of trainees first gathers, trainees should be asked to make a brief speech about their profession, where they work, and what they hope to get out of the training program. Knowing a trainee's therapy context (i.e., where he or she works or teaches) is important because it has considerable influence on how the training is received.

The supervisor should make a short speech at the beginning of the training period explaining how the training will be conducted and emphasizing issues of responsibility.

The supervisor can tell the trainees that they should each interview in their accustomed way and that he or she will correct them if their style differs much from the approach used in the training program. Otherwise, trainees will not use their previous experience in the interview room and may sit immobile, trying to guess what the supervisor might wish them to do. It is recommended that trainees avoid two kinds of behavior: making interpretations, particularly those relating the past to the present, and those emphasizing the usual negative motives; and they should not ask family members how they feel. If these interventions are avoided, the information from, and opportunities with, the family will be surprisingly improved, and the trainees will feel—and be—more effective.

By the end of the first training session the trainees should be looking forward to the next one. By then they should be acquainted with the facilities and procedures of the training program as well as with the basic rules of the therapy, as presented in a brief seminar, and they should have had the opportunity to express their desires and concerns about the training program.

A supervisor should, of course, know how to teach ways to do a first interview with a family, an individual, and a couple. Therapy is a skill which can be taught, and, like any skill, it must be learned with practice. Of course, human beings and their problems are remarkably complex, and there are as many ways of changing people as there are healers in the world. Yet the issues must be discussed and simplified, and theoretical positions must be taken.

A useful teaching device today is the videorecording of sessions. A supervisor can accumulate training tapes that demonstrate different ways to do a first interview, to motivate a client to follow a directive, to give the directive, to deal with the client's reaction, and so on. When videotapes are routinely made of trainee sessions, they become a mine of information and a valuable resource for demonstrating clinical skills.

GATHERING INFORMATION

Before a first interview the supervisor should provide the therapist with certain information, which is usually obtained from the client on the telephone, sometimes by a secretary and sometimes by a therapist. Certain facts, including the age and occupation of the client (or of the parents if it is a case involving a child), should be obtained. It is important to find out who lives in the household and the ages of the children. If there is a divorce, one needs to know who has custody of the children. During the initial phone call the client should be asked for a brief statement of the problem. A full discussion is to be avoided, but a simple statement of the problem (e.g., "A marital problem," or "My daughter keeps running away," or "My son is a drug addict") is helpful.

It is important to know whether there has been previous therapy, and, particularly, whether another therapist is currently involved. If insurance is available, what kind is it? The name and/or position of the person who referred the client is important since that person might have to be contacted. Sometimes a person is in distress and is sent from a crisis center. Sometimes a school refers a child who is having difficulty. Sometimes a case involves drugs or sexual abuse or violence, and therapy is court ordered and therefore is compulsory therapy. Sometimes a former client makes the referral, which is nice.

It is important to know whether a client is in therapy with someone else because the therapist's position in the hierarchy of colleagues is a basic concern. For example, if child protective services is referring a case, what is the legal situation? If the client is on medication, how much power does the prescribing physician have in the situation? It is best for the supervisor to protect the trainee from colleagues and to clarify the limits of the trainee's authority in the case.

One should not teach the taking of a social history or a genogram of an individual or family. Although this can be taught more easily than how to do therapy and may help beginners and supervisors start the training process, it defines therapy in ways one would rather not. For example, it teaches that therapy is about the past when, in fact, the therapy will focus on the present and the future. The client's social situation should be explored in the action of the interview, not separately.

It usually saves time to ask that everyone who lives in the household come to the first interview. However, if the caller wishes to be seen alone or if there seems to be such bad feeling that a whole family interview would be noxious, the caller can be interviewed alone. Generally, the client shouldn't be the one who determines who comes to the therapy sessions. That is a professional decision.

HOW TO OPEN THE FIRST INTERVIEW

A first interview with an individual requires different clinical skills of the therapist than one with a couple or a whole family. What an individual tells a therapist in body movements or in words is in relation to the therapist, not others, even if comments are about others. What a man says to a therapist when he is seen alone is probably not what he would say in the presence of his mother.

There are three ways that clients communicate with their therapist. They choose a position in the room in relation to the therapist and family members; they communicate with body movement; and they use words, in all their complexity and potential for multiple meanings.

Position is important. A client may sit close to the therapist or far away. Parents might sit with a child between them, which may indicate that the child has that function. A child might sit far away from other family members as a way of indicating that he or she is not involved. A couple can sit near each other, indicating that they are a unit, or sit turned away from each other. All of these various ways of positioning are influenced by cultural differences but are also a comment on the individuals and their response to the therapy situation. While the same positions might have other meanings at home or in different social situations, in therapy it's best to assume that clients are conveying information by the ways they move and sit. For example, an adult who is in the therapy room reluctantly will let the therapist know that, and his or her way of communicating should be respected.

Trainees must be taught by the supervisor to assume that all messages in the therapy room are to the therapist and are not merely a report about the client's state. For example, if a client is too anxious to sit down, this is not merely a report about his or her inner state but a message to the therapist. The more indirect the message, the more the person is indicating that he or she doesn't know the therapist and so doesn't know how the therapist will receive and respond to him or her. If the therapist says something and the client turns away slightly, it may be that the client won't risk a more direct comment at this time.

Supervisors should teach that it is a grave error to comment directly on or interpret a client's body movement. If a therapist says, "Have you noticed that you looked away when I said that?" the person will consider the therapist naive and/or rude, though he or she might not say so. From then on the person will not know how to move for fear the therapist will comment again and take any movement personally.

Since therapists want their clients to tell them those things that are often difficult to talk about, they must make it as easy and safe as possible. If a client expresses something in body movement, the therapist should accept that communication (if the client wished to translate the metaphor, he or she would do it).

It is often a new experience for a family to sit down together and talk, particularly about a family problem. Most families don't even have dinner together these days. It's especially unfamiliar to talk about one's problems with a stranger. Clients don't know how they are expected to behave and should be given some guidance. Even if they've had previous therapy, they're still not experienced in talking with this therapist and may be unfamiliar with the particular approach. For example, a client who was asked to express feelings by a previous therapist can become emotional during a first interview and the trainee may misunderstand, thinking this is the nature of the client when in fact it may only be what the client thinks the trainee wants. It helps to say something like, "I want everyone to say what is on their mind, and to take turns listening to each other."

A supervisor should teach a trainee the first steps in making everyone in the client's family comfortable. As family members take off their coats and seat themselves, it's helpful if the therapist makes small talk such as, "Did you have trouble finding the place" or "Isn't the traffic awful?"

If the therapy room has a one-way mirror and video cameras, the supervisor must teach trainees how to introduce these. One way is to say, "The way we work here is this: We have a one-way mirror and I have a colleague or colleagues behind it who might call in on this telephone and make suggestions. Two heads are better than one. These are video cameras, and I am taping the sessions because I like to see the interview later and see what I missed. At the end of the session, I'll ask you to sign a release. If you don't wish to sign, I'll erase the tape."

The more matter-of-factly the mirror and cameras are introduced, the more acceptable they are. Sometimes there are questions like, "You mean there is someone behind that mirror?" and "Why doesn't the person come in here?" An answer like, "That's the way we work," is often best.

Clients can be hesitant about talking about a problem and it's important not to let the introduction to the special features of the room take precedence over dealing with why they are there. Most clients have no objection to the arrangement that facilitates observation by the supervisor and other therapists. If a client seriously objects to being taped or observed, the drape can be drawn covering the mirror and the cameras can be turned off. A truly suspicious person can be taken to another room without such equipment. This is quite rare, but the client has the right to avoid being observed or filmed. Because training usually requires observation, the client who refuses to allow it sometimes must be transferred to a therapist who is not in training. The supervisor should make these final decisions, not the trainee.

The opening of the first interview should make the family feel as comfortable as possible. The therapist, while being an expert, should be a nonthreatening, benevolent presence, not distant and neutral but personal and friendly. This is a difficult time for a client, and therapists should use all their personal style to make it easy for them to talk. A question to the children as well as the parents, is helpful. The therapist can begin by asking, "What school do you go to?" or "What grade are you in?" or even "What did you expect in coming here?" The idea is to make it clear that everyone will be involved in the therapy. It may be useful for the trainee to see videotapes of family interviews as a way of preparing for the encounter.

Often clients wonder about qualifications, particularly if the therapist is young, and may ask, "Are you a doctor?" or "What is your profession?" Answers should be brief to indicate expertise, such as, "I'm a licensed social worker," or "I'm a clinical psychologist." Trainees who are asked if they are in training should acknowledge that they are by saying, for example, "I'm a therapist, and I am here for special training in the approach used here."

Sometimes a mother will ask, "Are you married?" or "Do you have children?" Trainees should answer briefly and frankly: "I'm not married," or "Yes, I am, and I have two children." These answers seem obvious, but many therapists have been taught confusing ways to answer personal questions because of strange theories about something called "transference." Generally, the therapist should allow personal questions, answer them briefly, and get on with the purpose of the meeting. A client has a right to check on the therapist's background but should not use the inquiry to avoid getting to the problem.

Sometimes, particularly if the parents are upset, a child will misbehave and interfere with the beginning of the therapy. The parents often don't know whether they should deal with the child or whether the therapist should. Therapists differ on this, as in many other matters, and supervisors should respect the therapist's opinion. Some like to deal with the child themselves. Others see this as an opportunity to gather information about the family and ask the parents to deal with the child in their usual way. If a parent hits a child, the therapist must object and say that other means of restraint need to be used. It is helpful to have a waiting room where small children can play while the parents are interviewed at the beginning stage of therapy.

If the presenting problem is a child, the supervisor should have the trainee expect to see the child alone. Most parents don't believe a therapist can evaluate a child in their presence, and assume that a therapist who sees the child alone is behaving like a child therapy expert.

With a couple or a family, the supervisor should teach the trainee how to determine who should be asked about the problem. This is a hierarchical issue. As an expert the family has called upon, the therapist has the authority to say who and what is important. When grandparents are in the therapy room, it might be respectful to ask them first about the problem. However, if the problem is a child and the therapist begins the interview by asking a grandparent about the problem, the therapist is essentially ignoring the parents' authority over the child; it might be better to focus on the parents and assign the grandparents the role of advisers. There are, however, exceptions to this solution: For example, the grandparents might have been given custody of the child by the court because of the parents' abuse of drugs; in that case the therapist should respect the fact that the grandparents have authority over the child, and therapy will deal with that issue.

If both parents accompany a child with a problem to therapy (and grandparents are not present), the therapist must decide which parent to ask for a description of the problem—and, consequently, which parent should be recognized as the authority. Typically, the mother is the prime caretaker, even in this age of women working, and she wants to define the problem. At times the father is quite involved, but he often seems to be a peripheral figure. To get a father more involved, the trainee can ask him about the problem. He will often pass the question on to his wife. At times a father is in a covert coalition with the child against the wife; asking him to define the problem gets to the issues more quickly.

If the child with a problem lives with a single parent, the trainee should look for another adult who is involved. Often the interview is with a single mother who lives with her mother. The therapist must be especially courteous to the grandmother while supporting the mother as the authority over the child. For example, the therapist can say to the grandmother, "I'll ask your daughter about the problem, and then I want to hear what you advise." Such a statement clarifies their relationship.

Often it is in a later interview that a single mother is joined by the grandmother or ex-husband or boyfriend, if that individual is important in the child's life. The therapist should spend a little time alone with the newcomer to help equalize the relationships.

With marital issues, the question is whom to ask what the problem is. If the therapist begins by asking the wife about the problem, she's likely to criticize the husband in a way that's difficult for him to recover from. Yet if one asks the husband about the problem, he's likely to pass it to his wife with a comment that minimizes the problem, a comment his wife may feel obligated to criticize.

Trainees need to try different ways to deal with this issue. Supervisors should teach them that the goal is to prevent both husband and wife from making comments that cause an irreversible break. Sometimes the therapist can begin the interview by asking, "If I asked your husband [or wife] what the problem is, what would he [or she] say?" The issue is always hierarchical.

The therapist has the power to influence who is higher in a marriage or in a parent–child relationship. The problem clients present will be related to some confusion in the hierarchy, and the ways a client presents it can be interpreted as a bid to form a coalition with the therapist. For example, if an adolescent daughter is threatening suicide, the parents will often surrender their authority and the adolescent will be in charge of what happens. The trainee, concerned about the suicide threat, is likely to defer to the adolescent and must be taught to step into the situation and reconstruct a correct hierarchy by joining in coalitions on all sides. The art of therapy is to join all sides in conflict with each other.

The task of a first interview is to define a solvable problem and start a change. This can only happen if the therapist organizes the interview. The therapist must take charge to change a problem. By the end of the first interview, the client should accept the therapist as the authority in the therapy.

HOW TO GAIN POWER

Two ways for the therapist to gain authority are (1) to decide who talks and (2) to decide what will be talked about. The therapist must invite everyone involved to speak, and he or she must organize that process. Even if family members talk together to resolve an issue, it should be done under the therapist's guidance. Therapists can take charge either by being central or by setting up a situation and then remaining on the sidelines while it is carried out.

What will be talked about must also be determined by the therapist. Whoever classifies topics is in charge. Clients appreciate being able to examine a life situation in new, more positive ways because their ways haven't worked. It is necessary for someone to take charge and offer assistance. Taking charge should not be tyrannical but subtle and inoffensive, so that resistance is not aroused. By listening to each person in turn, thus gratifying each client, the therapist establishes the fact that he or she is organizing the meeting. This is further confirmed if the therapist can later summarize what is said in a practical way and have it accepted.

With a proper first interview the individual or family will feel understood, will find the therapist benevolently concerned about each of them, will consider the therapist competent to deal with their problems, will find that hope has been generated, and will be accepting of some hierarchical changes—and the trainee and supervisor should be pleased with their own collaboration.

MAKING A THERAPY PLAN

Talking with a trainee about the information on the intake sheet is the beginning of what is sometimes a difficult task for the supervisor. The task is to plan the first interview in terms of what can be expected—but in such a way that the trainee will be able to drop the plan if it proves inappropriate when the interview takes place. Some trainees have been taught that it's wrong to plan, that they should approach the interview without any preconceived notions about the direction it should take. It is recommended here that the supervisor and therapist plan as much as they can. If the plan proves not to be appropriate, it can be dropped and another plan instigated. Often the planning is done in front of the group of trainees as a way to educate the group. The discussion is between the supervisor and the therapist who is about to do the interview, but the discussion can be opened up at times to the group for their ideas.

Let's suppose a client family has arrived and is in the waiting room. Examining the intake sheet, the therapist learns that there is a mother in her 40s, a stepfather slightly younger, a 16-year-old daughter, and a 12-year-old son. The presenting problem is "My daughter keeps running away." There are two tasks for the supervisor: (1) how to resolve the problems of this family and (2) how to teach the trainee how to think about and deal with such problems (what a supervisor might take for granted as he or she surveys a new clinical situation for the first time may be routine for some trainees and completely new to others and must be explicitly stated).

A first question is: Who should be brought into the interview room? Should it be the whole family? Should the daughter be seen alone first, or should the parents be seen alone first without the children? The decision of whom to interview first is based on the therapist's ideas about the presenting problem.

The daughter who is running away might be running from something or running to something. If she's running from something, there might be abuse in the home. Since the father is a stepfather, perhaps the triangle between the mother, stepfather and daughter is too intense. Perhaps the stepfather is sexually abusing the girl, and she is running away from that. If she is running *to* something, it might be a boyfriend or a group of friends. It's typical of a runaway adolescent girl to be running to a boyfriend the parents don't approve of. Parents have the problem of encouraging their children to have friends but not certain friends. When there is a problem, the daughter typically has chosen a boyfriend who is much older, who is a member of an ethnic group the parents disapprove of, or who has problems of some kind, such as an addiction to alcohol or drugs.

This speculation suggests that it is the daughter who should be seen first. If she is abused, she might reveal this if she is interviewed alone (but probably not if her parents are present). Yet if the therapist starts by seeing the daughter alone, the parents, who have been left in the waiting room, will wonder what she's revealing about the family. Since an obvious goal of therapy with a child out of control is to empower the parents, the therapist doesn't wish to undermine their authority. Listening to their daughter first while they are kept waiting and don't know what she's saying can do that. In this case it was decided to see the whole family together first and to see the daughter alone later on to inquire about private issues.

In the discussion with the trainee, the supervisor should clarify how a position must be taken on the following variables:

Problem. The therapy should focus on the presenting problem (in this case, the daughter's running away).

Unit. The unit of observation and intervention is the triangle. (In this case, the triangle of mother, and stepfather, and daughter is the basic unit of the problem, although other relevant triangles may be mapped in the family.)

Sequence. It is assumed that there are sequences that keep repeating in the family (here, the daughter's running away is an attempt to change the sequence but also keeps the sequence going).

Hierarchy. The structural focus is on the hierarchy in the family. (In this case it is assumed that the daughter has more power than the parents in determining what happens. By running away and risking harm to herself, she causes the parents to capitulate when there is a disagreement with her. To empower the parents the therapist must side with them whenever possible. This raises the issue of whether a young trainee therapist might have difficulty joining the parents against a problem adolescent since there may be a generational pull toward a coalition with the girl against the parents. If the therapist is older, he or she might feel a temptation to side with the parents. It is the supervisor's task to anticipate a trainee's personal biases and deal with them.)

Motivation. The hypothesis chosen to explain the motivation of the girl for running away is crucial. It is best for the supervisor to teach that adolescent misbehavior has some positive function in the family. Thinking this way in this case helps the therapist to consider the girl as helpful and not just a problem. An extreme view is that she can be thought of as a cotherapist, since she is misbehaving to *help* the family.

Keeping these variables in mind, the therapist will think of the young woman as in a triangle with her parents, will focus on her running away as the problem, will try to determine its positive function and change the sequence involved, and will attempt to empower the parents. The therapist must learn to join the parents while also joining the daughter.

By the end of the planning session the supervisor should have focused on the problem, expressed concern about the triangle with the stepfather, emphasized the need to empower the parents and correct the hierarchy, and conveyed to the trainee that the daughter is achieving something positive by running away. The personal biases of the therapist will have been noted by the supervisor without comment; these can be changed more successfully after the therapy begins rather than in a discussion dealing with hypotheses.

Given the information about this family before the session, the therapist can expect to find that there are difficulties surrounding the integration of the stepfather into the family. The integration of a stepparent into a family is becoming a national task. Due to a 50% divorce rate stepparenting is becoming more and more common. Supervisors need to have a way of doing something about the problems involved. It is a stage of family life that some couples can't get past. Usually the husband is too hard on the children because he thinks his wife is too lenient with them. She thinks he, not realizing how vulnerable they are, is too hard on them and she tries to restrain him. It is the supervisor's task to help the trainee end this sequence. The mother needs to be persuaded that she should encourage her husband to behave like a parent, despite her concerns. Often, she needs to be seen alone for this discussion. The husband needs to modify the ways he deals with the children so that his wife won't become upset. Of course, there are other alternatives, such as having the stepfather behave like a kindly uncle and not discipline the children at all. Each couple can work out their own satisfactory was of handling this situation.

It's possible that the daughter's problem behavior, that is, her running away, is an attempt on her part to integrate the stepfather in to the family. If this is so, the supervisor should teach the trainee how to support the stepfather's integration into the family so that the daughter will no longer need to resort to her own way of attempting to accomplish this goal.

Sample Case 1

The case under discussion is, in fact, not a hypothetical one but an actual therapy situation that I videotaped and use in training. The therapist was David Eddy, who was executive director of my institute at that time.

When the family, who were white, came in for their first interview, it was found that the daughter had been running away to join an African American boyfriend and stay at his house with his mother. Her mother and stepfather didn't approve of the young man. The family had actually resolved most of its problems when they came in for therapy. The girl was back at home, and she and her parents had agreed on the following issues: She could stay out in the evening until the hour she and her parents had selected; she could go out with the boyfriend; she could stay out of school that semester (since she was so far behind), but she had to find a job and was expected to return to school in the fall.

The crises that had brought the family to a therapist was a fight the mother and daughter had in the street when the daughter refused to come home. After the fight the mother had taken the daughter and dumped her with her biological father (the therapist and supervisor learned of his existence in this initial interview). The daughter was unhappy with her father and wanted to come back home to her mother. The mother and stepfather agreed to let her come back on certain terms, which led to the negotiations. The mother was allowing the stepfather to make decisions about the daughter, and in that sense the stepfather was integrated into the family. (In fact, the stepfather revealed in this interview that he was planning to adopt the children.)

The therapist and supervisor faced a dilemma in this case. The goal was to have the daughter stop running away, to empower the parents to be in charge of her, and to integrate the stepfather. The parents came in with a plan that they and the daughter had agreed to, yet it wasn't a good plan. Expecting the girl to find a job at age 16 and with no transportation was unrealistic. Nevertheless, the therapist's opposition to this plan would have undermined the parents, who had already negotiated this arrangement with the daughter. The therapist and supervisor decided to go along with what the parents had agreed to. The girl ended up working in her mother's office, and the parents accepted the boyfriend in their home for dinner (which was quite a concession for them). At that point the daughter began to be interested in a boy in the office.

The first therapy interview followed the plan, which was to focus on the daughter's running away, on integrating the stepfather into the family, and on empowering the parents so that the daughter followed their rules. It was hypothesized that running away helped the family in various ways: (1) The daughter made so much trouble that the mother had to let the stepfather take more responsibility as a parent, and (2) the biological father was moved further to the periphery of the family than in the past, which allowed the stepfather more room to assume the role of the father. There was yet another way the daughter helped: The mother had a sister who had married an African American man after a family uproar. In fact, the mother wasn't on speaking terms with her sister. When the daughter took up with this young man, the mother began to communicate with her sister. Thus, the daughter was instrumental in reuniting her mother and her aunt.

The family was followed by the therapist but was seen irregularly.

The therapist made no major interventions but simply supported what the family had worked out. The young woman didn't run away again, and she returned to school in the fall, as she had agreed.

There are typical family structures and problem hierarchies that can be anticipated when dealing with cases that involve child and adolescent problems. The situations are not so typical when a case involves a marital couple or an individual client; often there is not enough information on the intake sheet for the therapist to use to make a plan. Still, there are a few obvious patterns that supervisors can teach trainees that can help them in devising a therapy plan.

Sample Case 2

A 25-year-old woman who lived with her mother reported on the telephone that she was anxious and had incapacitating panic attacks.

The supervisor suggested to the trainee assigned to the case that the situation could be thought of as follows: The focus should be on the symptom, the problem would be found to be a triangle, there would be a problem hierarchy, and it would be found that the young woman was helping someone with her symptom. The initial interview was planned to explore these variables.

At the first interview, the young woman proved to be quite attractive and extremely nervous. She asked that the interview room door be left open in case she needed to get up and leave. She also declined to sit down and stood by the open door. In this way she, and not the therapist, was determining how the therapy would be conducted. (As is typical, the client was using her symptom to influence the hierarchy in the therapy situation.)

The therapist, Randy Fiery, remained standing and talked with the client patiently. After a while he sat down, and the young woman did also. He then suggested shutting the door so that they could talk privately (he indicated that she could sit close to the door if she wished to). She agreed.

The woman then explained that she had been living by herself in an apartment after breaking up with her boyfriend. She had been the manager of a retail store. When she quit because of her anxiety, her employer tried to persuade her to stay, which suggested that she was competent.

A few weeks prior to the interview the client began to have such severe panic attacks that she left her apartment and moved in with her mother, who had been living alone (the parents had been divorced for several years). As the therapist explored the triangle between mother, father, and daughter it became evident that the client was caught between her parents, who hadn't spoken to each other for 7 years. Whatever business they needed to transact with each other was done by using the daughter as an intermediary. In the past the daughter had alternately lived with each parent until she got her own apartment, which for her was a big step toward independence. Now she was once again the communication link between her father and mother. The client also reported that her mother had a drinking problem and that she was trying to help her mother stop drinking.

By the end of the first interview the therapist and supervisor had focused on the symptom (the anxiety) and had explored the triangle with the parents; it seemed evident that the daughter, in trying to be helpful to her parents, was sacrificing her own life. The mother was invited to the next interview, and she accepted.

She expressed irritation with her daughter for trying to run her life and for trying to get her to drink less. She said that she couldn't get her daughter to mind her own business. The daughter admitted that she couldn't help herself because of her anxiety. The mother complained that her place was too small for her daughter to be staying with her and felt that her daughter should be working. The mother was angry at the father and always had been. When the therapist suggested that the daughter would be less anxious if mother and father came together for an interview, the mother protested. Finally, she agreed. However that evening she called the therapist and said that she just couldn't stand being in the same room with her ex-husband.

When the daughter was next seen alone, she discussed her boyfriend, who had beaten her, and mentioned that she had been sexually abused by her paternal grandfather. Therapist and supervisor felt it was an opportunity to bring the parents together because of the issue of sexual abuse. By making an issue of the sexual abuse, the therapist was giving the mother and father an excuse to come in with the daughter. The daughter described her grandfather's fondling of her as a child. Her father said that he didn't remember such an event. Mother said, "You should. You spoke to your mother about it at the time." As the interview continued, the mother and father talked with each other about different family issues. At the end of the interview they said they were willing to meet again.

The therapist encouraged the young woman to reapply for her managerial position. She did so and was rehired. It proved helpful when the therapist encouraged her to do a body image appraisal of herself; with his help she discovered her attractive features. Her anxiety decreased. She came in for therapy with her mother, and they were able to straighten out some issues between them. The mother began to drink less, perhaps as a result of her improved relationship with her daughter.

Another interview with both parents freed the daughter of being a conduit for communication between them: Afterward, mother and father began to talk on the telephone.

The young woman dropped her anxiety and focused on problems of living. She was fond of her therapist and found him sympathetic and trustworthy. Without that personal trust, interventions rarely achieve their goals.

This example is used to show how a supervisor and therapist can think about a problem as a social event even when the problem is a symptom like anxiety. The directives given by the supervisor were essentially coaching directives, which is one of class of straightforward directives.

THERAPIST RELAPSE

It sometimes happens that a therapist "relapses" after training—that is, the therapist reverts to an inappropriate therapy approach in a particular case. For example, a therapist might be providing directives to a client and finds that the client doesn't follow any of them. In exasperation the therapist scolds and chastises the client, even blaming him or her for the therapy not going well. This behavior indicates a relapse on the part of the therapist to the orientation that people are rational and that they can be transformed if one explains to them how they are not behaving as they should. This assumption should be corrected and dealt with by the supervisor. There are also therapists who relapse after obtaining a job in a situation, such as an inpatient residential program, where brief and active therapy cannot be done.

A more serious relapse is the one that occurs after training is over. The relapsed therapists return to the ways of doing therapy that they learned before undergoing training for brief, directive therapy. I remember a young therapist who came to train with me and was interested in learning a variety of therapy approaches. He was bright and flexible and did quite well working in a brief approach with his cases. He also undertook some special training with me in treating young schizophrenics and their families. He was successful with a difficult case, and his future as a skilled therapist seemed assured.

Several years later I decided to make a training film that included this young man's successful therapy with a young woman who had been diagnosed schizophrenic. I visited him to get his permission to put his name in the film. When I told him I wished to make this film, he asked me not to. He said he now had a quiet private practice of long term therapy with clients who came in on time, paid their bills, and had no crises. He no longer wanted to treat difficult cases. He said that if his name was put in the film, other therapists would refer crazy and difficult clients to him, and that he did not want to deal with such clients and their families anymore.

I did not release the film. I regretted the time I had spent teaching this young man a brief and effective therapy with difficult cases. He would never use that knowledge or pass it on to others. Supervisors must live with such relapses.

10

MORE ON DIRECTIVES

TELLING PEOPLE WHAT TO DO

There is a common misunderstanding about directive therapy. One doesn't give directives only to bring about change. One gives a directive to establish a type of relationship. Rather than talk about past causes or the client's childhood experiences, action is generated in the present by discussing the directive. The approach is similar to Zen Buddhism, where it has some of its origins. Rather than talking to a student about the past or about his or her emotional life a Zen Master gives a task. For example, the master teaches the art of swordsmanship or of flower arranging, and that becomes the subject of discussion with the trainee. Enlightenment occurs from that involvement. In the same way, giving a directive and discussing the response is the action of directive therapy.

Among the ways to classify directives is to say that some are straightforward. One simply tells the client what to do. Other directives are indirect, as when one restrains the client from changing or encourages a symptom. In the same way, the directives used in training a therapist can be classified as straightforward or indirect. The choice of which type of directive to use can be based on the therapist's power. Usually, indirect approaches are used with a client when straightforward directives aren't followed. This also happens between supervisor and therapist. When the supervisor has sufficient authority the trainee does what he or she is told. When that authority is insufficient, indirect techniques can be used.

For example, if it is necessary in order to deal with a problem that a trainee asks a client couple about their sex life but the trainee avoids doing so, the supervisor can direct the trainee to ask the couple certain questions. If the trainee is unable to ask such questions about the couple's sex life—that is if he or she keeps beginning to ask these questions and then drifts away from the subject—then a more indirect approach may be needed. The supervisor apparently doesn't have the authority to persuade the trainee directly.

Straightforward Directives

Typical straightforward directives include telling a person what to do, offering advice, coaching step by step, setting up an ordeal, or establishing a penance. These contrast with influencing the person with metaphor, or doing nothing until the person takes action spontaneously.

Straightforward directives to a trainee typically involve learning interview skills. For example, let's say that a trainee gets into a one-to-one conversation again and again in a family interview. He talks to the mother, and then to the father, and then to the child. Whenever he's talking to one of the family members, the others sit back and wait until he's done. They don't spontaneously participate. Often this one-to-one style of interviewing is a result of previous experience doing therapy with individuals. The trainee is more comfortable talking with one person rather than several at once. The supervisory problem is that the family does not talk with each other but with the therapist, and so must have the therapist present to discuss an issue. The supervisor watching behind the mirror can find him- or herself thinking that with this individual focus the other family members might as well be in the waiting room.

A straightforward way to deal with this problem is to discuss it with the therapist and to point out that the interview should be done differently. The therapist should ask the mother about the father, and the father about the mother, and either one about the child. That is a way of activating their relationships with each other. After such a discussion, the supervisor can guide the therapist on the telephone from behind the mirror. When the mother says she is upset, the therapist should turn to the father. If he doesn't, but continues with the mother, the supervisor can call and suggest asking the father if he knows why his wife is upset. The father makes a comment and the wife disagrees or wishes to correct him. She will do so when free to talk to her husband and not just to the therapist. As the therapist talks through one family member to another, they begin interchanges, which can be helpful and productive. The therapist becomes less necessary, which is the goal of the therapy, and the supervisor becomes less necessary, which is the goal of the training.

This seems a simple instruction and sometimes it is, but making such a change can be a problem for some therapists when their interviewing style expresses the ideology of individual therapy. The supervisor not only has to call in each time to get such therapists to do what they should, but he or she might have to bring such therapists out of the room and review with them again how they should be talking through the family members to each other. This directive to the therapist is a straightforward one; the supervisor is essentially coaching the trainee.

Directives for Clients Who Make Long Speeches

An example of a one-to-one situation is when parents make a long speech about a child's problem. Some parents with a problem adolescent start with the child's first cold and take the therapist through year after year of childhood experiences. Other family members begin to doze off in boredom. Often the parent has rehearsed the speech the night before the interview to be sure to fully inform the therapist. Trainees may have difficulties with this when they have been taught to be courteous with families and think it is rude to redirect a parent's focus. If the trainee says, "The past is not important; it's the present that's the issue," the parent may be offended and may assume the therapist doesn't understand the full extent of the problem. The parent will then go on at even greater length to educate the therapist for the remainder of the interview.

Correcting usually doesn't help and can antagonize a parent. Moreover, trying to redirect a client by summarizing often leads to the client's correcting the summary at length. The standard supervision procedure in this situation is to teach the trainee to turn to another family member when the opportunity arises. When one parent takes a breath, the therapist can turn to the other parent and ask if he or she has the same opinion as the spouse. Or the therapist can turn to the child and ask him to listen to the loquacious parent to be sure he or she understands the parent's objections. This can lead to a conversation with the child. The goal is to escape the past and get into action in the present as quickly, and as politely, as possible.

I recall Milton Erickson dealing with a family in which the mother talked and did not let the other family members speak. She would say what they would have said if they had had the chance, but she never let them have the chance. Erickson said to the woman, "I don't believe you can hold your thumbs a quarter inch apart." "Of course I can do that," said the woman, and she put her thumbs within a half inch of each other. "I'm sure you can't continue to do that," said Erickson. "Certainly I can," she replied. Erickson said, "While you do that, I'll ask the others some questions, and I want you to listen carefully because I want you to have the last word." He then talked with the youngest boy, and then the older one, and then the father. When the mother started to disagree, Erickson would point to her thumbs, which moved when she spoke. She would reposition her thumbs and resume the silence confined by the directive because it was so absurd.

If the supervisor is less innovative and prefers a more moderate approach, telephoning the therapist can be helpful in dealing with a parent who is dominating the conversation. That interruption quiets the family member, who must wait for the phone call to end, and it gives the therapist a chance for a fresh start. Telephoning is itself an intervention: It can interrupt a person's monologue as well as break up an unproductive sequence being followed by the family. With a really determined monologuist, the supervisor can phone a request to the therapist to step out of the room for a conference, which creates an even larger interruption. Such a tactic is also helpful when a long-winded client and a trainee who has just learned to listen to individuals meet each other.

I recall Virginia Satir saying she could determine whether a therapist was thinking in terms of systems theory by asking him or her to describe a case. She said that it took her less than five minutes to make the determination and that if she had watched the therapist work with a family, it would have taken her only three minutes. A therapist's behavior in an opening interview reveals the presence or absence of a systems view so the supervisor can see what needs to be taught.

Objections to Directives

There are two major principles of the directive approach that some therapists object to. One is that the therapist takes responsibility for what a client should do. These therapists prefer to explore and discuss. Sometimes it's helpful to point out to them that they can't avoid giving directives. If they don't tell the client what to do, they are saying, "Don't ask me what to do," which is a directive.

The other principle some therapists object to is that the directive therapist acknowledges that he or she is deliberately trying to influence the client. It helps to point out to these therapists that one can't avoid influencing the client and that one only has a choice about whether to acknowledge it or not. Carl Rogers is a good example. He argued that he wasn't telling clients what to do, that he only reflected back to them what they were saying.[1] However, Rogers didn't reflect everything back; he chose to reflect only certain ideas. By doing so he guided the client to the topics he felt should be talked about.

[1]Rogers, C. R. (1951). *Client centered therapy.* Boston: Houghton Mifflin.

Another problem some trainees have with directives is that they often feel they don't know what to do, and they don't know how to maintain their expert status, when a client doesn't follow the directive. Of course, it is the supervisor's task to teach them how to respond when clients don't follow directives. The same procedures that are taught can also be used when trainees don't do what the supervisor says. The first step is for supervisor and trainee to explore what the objections are. If the directive is, in fact, unsatisfactory, the next step is for the supervisor to apologize. Supervisors in this situation can misunderstand the clinical situation because if they had offered the correct procedure in the correct way the trainee would surely have followed the directive. Usually this either leads to the trainee following the directive or providing a better one. An apology is always powerful.

One reason to have trainees begin doing therapy at the beginning of the training, rather than read about it and do it later is because they're eager to have someone tell them what to do when faced with a client. Usually, beginning trainees follow their supervisor's directives without hesitation.

There is also an inherent inertia in some trainees that the supervisor must fight against. Therapy was easy when all a therapist had to do was know how to say, "Tell me more about that," or "I wonder why you did that." Therapists only needed to know how to converse with the client— and any adult has had years of practice conversing. To act and to bring about change means knowing what to do. Understandably, some trainees are hesitant about issuing directives to clients unless they are confident they are getting proper guidance.

INDIVIDUAL OR FAMILY INTERVIEW

In determining who is involved in a family's problem it's helpful for the therapist to think of the family in terms of triangles. For example, if a mother is being guided by a therapist to help her child, the therapist should suspect that there is a husband or grandmother or other adult who is also involved and should consider the possibility that that person might feel antagonized and might attempt to defeat the therapy if he or she is left out of it.

For example, a woman in her 20s, upset over breaking up with her boyfriend, attempted suicide by jumping off a bridge. Several bones were broken. She moved in with her mother and came to therapy. The therapist suggested that her mother come in, but the young woman said that that was unnecessary, that she was only going to live with her mother for a short time, and that she would then be on her own again. The therapist accepted the client's view. However, a few weeks later the young woman discovered that she was pregnant. She wished to keep the child. The therapist telephoned the mother to come in and make plans for her daughter. The mother flatly refused. She said that the therapist hadn't wanted her to be part of the therapy before and that the therapist could deal with the pregnancy without her now. The mother's refusal required the therapist to continue with the young woman and help her through the birth of her child, which might more appropriately have been done by the mother.

A trainee therapist must be taught that every client in individual therapy is related to someone. A wife might be seen alone, but the therapist must remain aware of the existence of her husband, who is part of the therapy even in he is not in the interview. A therapist can become fascinated with a client's ideas or perceptions and forget that other people are involved in what happens in that person's life. Just being in therapy is a response, as well as a message, to others.

It is difficult for a therapist to make a judgment on what to do when some family members refuse to come in for an interview. Family therapy is difficult enough without having to deal with the absence of a crucial participant. If the therapist believes failure will occur without certain family members in therapy, the obvious thing to do is drop the case. It is part of the bill of rights of therapists that one does not have to participate in failure. Or, one can start with part of the family and hope that the others will join the group later. Trainees must understand that often a family has been blamed by therapists in the past and doesn't wish to repeat the experience; such a family must be persuaded that this time will be different.

Shifting a trainee from seeing a family to seeing an individual alone should be a simple procedure, not an elaborate formal arrangement. The trainee must learn to determine who is to be seen and when, based on the recognition that a family member is holding something back because of the presence of other members. Seeing that person alone or even each family member alone, can bring out helpful information. When the supervisor senses a mystery, he or she can recommend that a family member be seen alone or that a different combination of family members be seen together. Since therapy sometimes starts with family members being excessively angry with each other it can be helpful to see them individually instead of beginning therapy with the whole family present.

There is always symmetry in human relations. If a mother is overinvolved with her child, her husband is likely to be overinvolved with someone else. If a man is too attached to a friend, his wife will become attached to someone else to balance that equation. Viewing a family this way, a therapist can anticipate the ways people are involved with each other. It can also be noted that the therapist is part of the balance. If a therapist is seeing a woman in individual therapy, the husband may become involved with someone else, sometimes a therapist of his own.

THE DESTINATION OF A SYMPTOM

Although doing a method therapy is too confining, supervisors in a brief, directive therapy training program can teach a number of helpful guidelines and procedures that can be used on different cases.

One procedure that is helpful to a therapist in formulating a problem is to have the client imagine the ultimate destination of a symptom. That is, the therapist can be taught to ask, "What if your problem gets worse?" Usually the client responds, "I will feel awful." One should pursue the issue further by asking, "And what if feeling awful gets worse?" As the therapist pursues the issue, the function of the symptom in relation to other people will become more evident.

I recall a case of a young woman with a trembling right hand. It shook irregularly and neurological tests failed to show a physical cause. She was referred to me for hypnosis. I asked her what would happen if the problem got worse. She said, "I'll lose my job." I asked, "And what if you lose your job?" She said, with a sigh, "My husband will have to go to work." Thus I found out that the woman had been supporting her husband, which she resented, and that her parents protested this arrangement to the point of trying to break up the marriage.

In pursuing the destination of a symptom, the therapist can sometimes get rid of it by making the destination explicit. For example, clients fear going mad from their symptom. When asked what will happen if their problem gets worse, they will say that they will go crazy. When the therapist asks them what will happen next, they say that they will go into a mental hospital and that that will be the end of the road. The therapist can point out that the person will be released on weekends, that with the reduction of hospital time for patients a permanent release will come in a few weeks, and that then the client will be sitting right there in the same chair and facing the same situation once again.

Consider yet another example of the utility of pursuing the destination of a symptom: A young man was arrested for possessing and dealing marijuana. He had been arrested several times and was recently referred to therapy. He was the youngest son and obviously the favorite. The therapist raised the issue with the family of what would happen if the young man relapsed and took drugs again. After a discussion about how disappointed they would feel, the family, with encouragement, realized that they themselves could set a severe consequence if the son relapsed. After a discussion the family decided to abandon their previous response to the son's behavior, that is, forgiving the young man each time he broke the law, in favor of a new response. As the therapist nicely put it, "The family decided that it could set a consequence if the son relapsed, or the community would do so by putting him in jail."

The therapist can also raise the question of what happens if a client's problem gets better. There are consequences and adjustments in a family when a member's chronic problem improves. If a man who has been a lifelong drinker stops drinking, the family has problems accepting the change. His wife has learned to do without him as a husband, and the children have to learn all over again that they must obey their father. Often, the husband has been replaced by an older son, who does not welcome the father's returning to power. Supervisors must teach trainees that change itself, not just failure, can be a problem

USING THE SELF IN THERAPY

Therapists can change their style, to some extent, but they cannot change their age, gender, or sometimes their profession. Supervisors must train therapists to take advantage of what they are. Generally, supervisors approach trainees with the intent to work within the trainee's style. (It seems inevitable that trainees will adopt much of the style of their supervisor, but that doesn't mean they become a carbon copy. Therapy training is an apprenticeship in an art, and artists often begin by adopting the ways of the master. As they develop their own ways and learn to use their own resources, the resemblance to the teacher disappears—except, one hopes, for the wisdom.) A trainee who responds slowly and leisurely does not need to be transformed into a rapid responder. Therapist's styles can vary, but each can accomplish what must be done. At times therapists must be authoritarian and tell clients what to do. At other times they need to appear helpless so that the client will take charge. However, each therapist can be authoritarian or helpless in his or her own way. The supervisor must not interfere with the essential nature of the trainee and need only ensure that the trainee has a style that allows a range of skills.

METAPHOR

As Intervention

It is in the area of change through metaphor that the question of who initiates the new behavior arises. This is why metaphoric interventions raise the most serious ethical questions.

In therapy everything is an analogy to something else. In fact, it is the nature of communication itself that messages are transmitted and received on multiple levels. (I recall during Gregory Bateson's research project in communication that we set out to make a dictionary of terminology. We decided to begin with the word "message." Then we added the word "metamessage" for messages about messages. We soon recognized that every message is a metamessage in that it qualifies some other communication.) If a parent says to a child, "Eat your dinner," the message isn't just about food. It's also about the parent–child relationship inasmuch as it expresses the idea that the child should do what the parent says, and because parents are nurturing. Whatever one says qualifies and is qualified by the situation in which it is said and has multiple meanings. Sometimes a metaphor is deliberately used in therapy and in training. If a supervisor describes a case to a trainee group, the case is an analogy containing ideas the trainee can use with other cases. It's a story with a moral, or a number of them. Every supervisor should have a collection of cases to illustrate different therapy interventions and premises about therapy. This book is just such an example.

The following is a description of a case of a deliberate metaphoric intervention: A father and a mother brought in a 12-year-old problem child who had been a problem for several years and had been through two unsuccessful therapies. He had a 10-year-old brother who was the golden boy of the family and had no problems. The therapist used family therapy and included the father. After the father became more involved with the child, the boy improved and began to do well at school.

At this point the mother said that since the boy had improved, she wanted to have the therapist improve their marriage. The therapist was willing, but the husband didn't want to discuss his marriage. He was there for the child, and that was that. The supervisor and therapist faced a problem: They could accept the father's position, finish therapy with the problem child, and leave an unhappy marriage; or they could argue with the father, a working class man who expressed himself with difficulty, and try to persuade him to discuss his marriage. Since his wife was articulate and more educated, the husband may have feared that she would put him down if he discussed his dissatisfaction with the marriage in therapy.

Another alternative was to improve the marriage without discussing it, but by using a metaphorical approach. The idea came about during live supervision: The mother was saying that the good child, the golden boy, was embarrassed by his brother's behavior, and it occurred to the therapist and supervisor that she seemed herself at times to have been embarrassed by the behavior of her husband. The mother was also saying that the problem boy couldn't talk as well as his brother could (just as her husband was less articulate than she). It seemed apparent to the supervisor, who was observing the clinical interaction from behind the one-way mirror, that to the mother the good boy was like her and the problem boy was like the father, and that it was possible to discuss the relationship between the two boys as metaphor for the relationship between the parents. Thus, the marital issues could be discussed without explicitly talking about the marriage. The supervisor telephoned to convey his idea. A trainee would have been called out of the therapy room to discuss this idea, but this was an experienced therapist and he quickly grasped the strategy. He began to ask the parents whether the two boys ever had good times together, whether they were able to resolve their difficulties, and so on. The couple immediately responded to this way of talking about the relationship of the two boys. Whether or not they realized that the discussion about their sons was a metaphor for a discussion of their own relationship is unknown. It is important when using this approach to prevent the participants' awareness of the metaphor. The use of metaphor must remain out of consciousness—or at least not be explicitly stated.

There is one other important intervention needed to bring about a change when using metaphor. Merely drawing the analogy between two relationships isn't sufficient. The therapist must take a position. In the case under discussion here the supervisor called and suggested to the therapist that he say what he thought the relationship between the boys should be. He did so, saying that the two brothers should enjoy spending time together and that each should also have time to himself. At this point the father began to talk about the importance of the problem boy having some time alone. In fact, he said without some time alone the boy would feel like a husband who comes home from work and immediately has all the problems of the day dumped on him by his wife instead of being able to relax with a beer and have some time to himself. The wife agreed a husband should be able to do the latter. It's interesting that the shift from the boy's relationship to a hypothetical marital one was made by the husband, the spouse who hadn't wanted to discuss marriage.

The next week the couple came in and reported that they had arranged for the father to have 20 minutes to himself when he comes home from work before he has to face the family's problems of the day. They apparently believed that this idea had come to them during the week. A series of similar changes were made in the marital relationship by talking with the couple about improving the relationship between their sons. Again, whether the couple knew that these discussions were metaphorical is unknown.

An ethical issue arises in this type of directive because the change is arranged outside the person's awareness, yet so much is gained by the richness of this approach that the ethical issues must be considered from that perspective.

Sanity and Madness

Metaphor can be used to change people, but there is another aspect of it that must be understood. Metaphor is also a type of communication one must respond to. A person who takes everything literally is handicapped and will miss most of the meaning of any communication in life. Every therapist must be trained to seek out the meaning a client is trying to communicate, and much of that meaning is embedded in metaphor and must be understood. For example, if a man is on trial and doesn't know what crime he has committed, he doesn't know what he might say that would prove him guilty. His safest course is to avoid direct communication and use metaphor, which can have multiple and ambiguous meanings. I recall a father who thought he was being blamed for his son's psychosis but had no idea of what he had done wrong. When he was asked a question about his son's condition, he wisely replied, "It's a certain species of something from somewhere else."

Metaphor is the basis of all art and religion. Metaphor is also the most emotionally loaded type of communication. It can lead to a life devoted to artistic creation. It can also lead to death by execution inasmuch as heresy may lie in the difference between a metaphor and a literal statement. One great heresy was whether the blood and body of Christ actually became bread and wine or only metaphorically. Many people died over that issue. Fortunately, such a consequence does not await the trainee therapist who confuses a metaphor with real life, but an awareness of that distinction is part of doing therapy. Therapists must learn something about the communication of dreams and fantasies and stories with a moral.

The most skillful people in the use of metaphor are those who are classed as schizophrenic. If a fellow says that he is from outer space, and seems to mean it, he becomes diagnosed as a special person who is in a difficult situation. If a man says he is Jesus Christ and really seems to believe it, he will be diagnosed as psychotic. Supervisors must teach trainees how to understand such communications. What should be taught? There are several options:

1. A person's use of metaphor can be taken to mean that the person has a thought disorder. Something is wrong inside the head of a man who says he was born on Mars. He is assumed to have a brain disease or a

neurological disorder, and therefore his statement is dismissed as a message about his inner condition, not a message *to* anyone. In this view, the goal becomes one of finding a drug to use to stop the person from talking in that disordered manner. The response is in terms of social control, not therapy.

2. The metaphor can be taken to mean that the person is communicating to someone—and doing it badly. His or her problem is a difficulty with those signals that indicate that he or she is speaking in metaphor. Such a person doesn't say, "It's like I was born on Mars," which would tell the listener that he or she came from a home which was like the home of the god of war, but instead "I was born on Mars." People who have difficulty using these signals also have difficulty when others use them. If a waitress says to such a person, "What can I do for you?" that person is sometimes uncertain what she has in mind and might respond deviantly.

3. A metaphor can also be used deliberately. If a man says he is Jesus Christ and sounds like he believes it, he may be offering the listener a choice in responding to him. The listener can respond as if he is speaking randomly or can take the self-description as a meaningful personal comment. If one accepts this assumption, it means accepting the idea that the person is deliberately using a metaphor and deliberately leaving out the indicators that it *is* a metaphor. He is communicating in a way that allows the person he is talking to an out and he need not notice that the comment is critical at a personal and organizational level.

What has this to do with therapy? It means that the supervisor must teach trainees to respect the communications of people diagnosed as schizophrenic and to listen to these metaphors for guidance in understanding the person's situation (while neither translating the metaphor nor speaking back in metaphor). If the trainee discusses the metaphor with the client, he or she will be like a novice chess player dealing with a master. The best way to respond is to focus on the simplest of ideas: Adult clients who are living at home should go to work or school and do what their parents say. They should be making plans to support themselves or to get training to do so. The trainee should be taught to be digital with people diagnosed as schizophrenic and their families, not analogic.

Of course this is an oversimplified way to discuss this complex problem. Obviously, various kinds of people get diagnosed as schizophrenic. However, trainees will have an advantage if they accept (but do not respond to) schizophrenic metaphor as a guide to understanding the client and focus on the most basic issues.

I recall the way John Rosen once reacted literally to a young man who said he was Jesus Christ: "Oh, you're the fourth Jesus Christ who came in today." With another he said, "If you stop claiming you're Jesus

Christ, I'll give you a new shirt." The young man cooperated and got the shirt.[2]

Sample Case

This section does not describe how to treat psychotics but how to think about seemingly psychotic comments in a therapy context. An 18-year-old woman began to run wild, and was placed on a psychiatric ward in a university hospital. When interviewed, she said she was pregnant with twin fetuses. Since she was menstruating at the time, her statement was taken as delusionary and indicating a thought disorder. She was brought out of the hospital with family-oriented therapy and went back to school and work, but she had an anticipated relapse when her parents threatened to separate.

In a family interview the young woman said she would kill herself if her parents separated because "those eight children need you." The young woman was acting strange in this interview and was insulting to the therapist. (It might be noted that it is typical for a young person who has relapsed to attack one parent and also the therapist, no matter how good these relationships previously were.) The supervisor, concerned about the threat of suicide if the parents separated, called the therapist out of the room. He asked the therapist if he could get angry at the girl. The therapist, having been insulted by her, thought he could. The supervisor suggested that the therapist say to the girl that she had no right to threaten her parents with suicide if they separated, and that they had the right to do what they felt was necessary, just as she did. Since the trainee was a intellectual type, he was encouraged to express his anger as a personal communication to the client and not simply as an intellectual observation. The trainee went back to the interview room, and after a few more insults from the girl, which helped, he managed to express his anger at her for taking away her parents' rights. One response to this came from the mother, who firmly told her daughter that whether she separated from her husband or not was not the daughter's business, that she would make the decision. From that point on the daughter began to behave more rationally in the interview and even joked with the therapist.

The metaphor of the twin fetuses was never discussed in the therapy of this case. It was accepted as meaning something about multiple births. That idea seemed an appropriate interpretation when it was found that the mother had had eight children and was exhausted and sad. When this daughter began to set out on her own life, the mother became depressed

[2]Rosen, J. N. (1951). *Direct analysis*. New York: Grune & Stratton.

and took to her bed. The daughter then began to act wild and to talk about multiple births. The trainee was advised to assume that the daughter understood her own metaphors and didn't need interpretations of them. The focus was on getting her back to school and work and resolving differences between her parents, not dwelling on her imaginative ideas.

The proper way for a trainee to respond to a young psychotic is to try to understand the metaphor but not necessarily to comment on its meaning. If the trainee does that, the client will express important ideas more and more freely. The client needs to be able to trust the therapist not to interpret or make accusations irresponsibly but, rather, to accept the ideas as part of a covert coalition until they can be expressed more explicitly. Trainees should be taught that not mentioning something they observe is not a sign of being dishonest but of being polite.

WHAT IS DISHONEST?

It is every supervisor's obligation to see to it that therapists-in-training do not learn to be dishonest. Typically, clients have been abused either physically, spiritually, or morally. They do not need to be deceived by a helping person. Dishonesty by a therapist isn't excused just because the therapist has good intentions. The question is: What is dishonesty? Is it dishonest to trick a client out of a symptom? For example, a person afraid of elevators was hypnotized by Erickson and sent to a certain address with the instruction to be totally concentrated on the soles of his feet. The address was, of course, a top floor in a tall building, and the client went up in an elevator to get there. He didn't realize he was in an elevator because he was fully focused on the soles of his feet. From then on he rode in elevators without fear. Was that intervention dishonest?

There is a situation that can arise when using paradox either with a client or with a trainee. The therapist is encouraging the person to have a symptom the therapist wishes the person to give up. Is that dishonest? As an example, a therapist was dealing with a 12-year-old boy who had for years masturbated in his living room in front of his sisters and mother. He had also masturbated at school. Two years of therapy hadn't improved this symptom. A supervisor arranged for the therapist to use a paradoxical approach. The boy was encouraged to masturbate in private and on Sundays, a day he had previously indicated was associated with the greatest masturbatory pleasures, but when he masturbated on other days, his punishment was that he had to do more of it on Sunday. The boy responded by masturbating less in public, and the therapist blamed him for not cooperating. There is typically a stage in the use of paradox where the client is partially improved and the therapist insists on the symptom.

This can be considered dishonest since the therapist is encouraging behavior he or she wishes to end. However, one can also think of this in a different way. Within the larger framework of the relationship, the therapist wants the person to get over the symptom. For example, in the case under discussion the therapist wants the boy to continue to masturbate, since this directive is part of the treatment. When one takes context into account, the question of honesty becomes complex: The therapist honestly wants the boy to masturbate—and not to masturbate. That's part of the paradox of the communication. It should be accepted that whether the client knows the therapist is using a paradox or not is not relevant. Awareness of what is being done is not the issue, and so it is not deceptive in that sense.

Once I was at a conference with a prominent therapist who had seen a videotape of the case of the masturbating boy. He said it was dishonest. The prominent therapist hadn't been trained in the use of paradox and had no experience with paradoxical techniques. Therefore, he did not understand the honesty issue in the way it is being presented here. Actually, paradox is at the heart of all therapy in the sense that the therapist must direct the client to change spontaneously.

Here is another case to illustrate the issue of dishonesty: A young woman was afraid of flying, a fear that was becoming more of a problem to her since she needed to travel for her job. She went to a psychiatrist and asked if he would use hypnosis to help her get over this symptom. At the end of the first session the psychiatrist said that he wished to see her in therapy for three months to deal with individual and family issues and that at the end of that time he would hypnotize her and rid her of her flying phobia. He said the three months of therapy were necessary to prepare her to recover. Since his fee was high, this meant there would be quite a financial investment from the young woman in this preparatory phase. Was the psychiatrist being dishonest and overcharging the young woman or was he being careful? What if he didn't know how to hypnotize anyone (most psychiatrists don't) and was assuming that after the woman was in therapy with him for three months the hypnosis would be unnecessary. It is the responsibility of the supervisor to define for trainees what is exploitation of a client, and therefore dishonest, and what is merely an issue of competence.

A NOTE ON SUPERVISING SUPERVISION

Years ago I was training therapists from the community who had no academic background. They became quite competent therapists, especially in dealing with the families of the poor, which was their specialty.

After they graduated, I discovered that they were being asked to teach because there were so few professional therapists who knew how to do family-oriented therapy. Since these therapists had been trained to be therapists, not to teach other therapists, they asked for help in learning how to teach.

That situation clarified for me some of the differences between teaching a therapist and teaching a teacher or supervisor. Therapists, professional or otherwise, do not necessarily need to conceptualize an ideology to do the work. They need to know what to do without necessarily being able to communicate the reasons for their actions to someone else. A teacher must pass on a way of thinking as well as a set of skills. Teachers of therapists have special requirements. Therapists must know how to treat their clients; teachers must know not only how to treat clients but also how to think about that action in ways that can be transmitted to others.

A supervisor today must be able to not only supervise therapists but also supervise supervisors. The tasks are different. A person who is a good supervisor of therapists might not be a good supervisor of supervisors. Many aspects are the same, but the teaching of teachers is a more intellectual enterprise. For one thing, the units are different: When supervising a therapist, the therapist and the client constitute the unit. When supervising a supervisor, the unit consists of the supervisor, the therapist, and the client; the extended hierarchy makes everything more complex. A simple idea proposed to a therapist to use with a client might be negated by a therapist unable to grasp it, or a supervisor-in-training may be unable or unwilling to transmit the idea. Sometimes, too, an idea from a supervisor to a supervisor to a therapist to a client undergoes many transformations along the way, and the client can sometimes end up with only a good intention.

Supervision of supervisors involves the usual problem of finding out what is actually happening in the therapy. It helps if the supervisor of a supervisor is behind the one-way mirror with him or her, in order to observe the interchange between the supervisor or therapist and the client. A problem in such a situation is that the therapist who comes out of the interview for consultation tends to orient hierarchically to the supervisor of supervisors and not to the supervisor. (One way I have tried to solve this is by supervising two supervisors at once in two different rooms. Each therapist becomes aware of my frequent absences, because I am observing events in the other therapy room, and so pays more attention to the supervisor-in-training who knows better than I what is happening.)

Going over video and audio recordings of therapy sessions or of supervision with therapists is also helpful when training a supervisor. The supervisor of supervisors can discuss the ways suggestions of supervisors are carried out by therapists, as well as some of the problems encountered in helping therapists who have particular difficulties. The problem with recordings, of course, is that one is talking about events that have passed, and guidance cannot occur at the moment of the action. However, since supervisors of supervisors deal with issues at a more strategic level, there can be a more general discussion, with the recording being used as a starting point.

Talking about a case from notes means working with the least information about what actually happens, but this, too, provides an opportunity for more general discussions about different kinds of interventions and the nature of different problems. Each case becomes a starting point for discussing various treatment options and directions for the particular kind of situation it exemplifies.

It is particularly important with case discussions that the supervisor-in-training present the case to his or her own supervisor. Not only do they share the same language and ideas, but the supervisor has already tried out the typical procedures used in such a case. The strategies used in similar cases have already been taught, and so the supervision discussion does not need to dwell on those possibilities. Assuming that routine procedures have already been tried, the supervisor can suggest new ideas for the supervisor-in-training that will expand his or her horizons. This kind of teaching is more of a burden on the supervisor of supervisors, because he or she must come up with ways of working and with ideas that are new to the supervisors-in-training.

The variables involved when supervising supervisors are the same as those involved when supervising therapists. In the discussion the focus is on the problems of the therapist. There are several typical aspects to such a discussion: (1) the attempt to find out how the therapist is involved with the client, (2) the search for new interventions that might help in a given case, (3) the correction of errors that might have been made by the therapist, and (4) the teaching of ideas that might be new to the supervisor-in-training and helpful with other cases. A case may also be a stimulus for a general discussion of the nature of therapy. There is freedom in such discussions to consider various therapeutic options, with the ultimate decision worked out later between the supervisor-in-training, the therapist, the client and family.[3]

THE RIGHT TEACHING CONTEXT

Whether training therapists or supervisors, it is important to arrange a setting that is appropriate for a brief, socially oriented therapy. The therapy field is in transition from a leisurely, exploratory therapy and supervision approach to an action-oriented way of working. Agencies are often continuing in traditional ways even as they try to change. It's the nature of agencies that there are bureaucratic procedures constructed upon the ideologies of the past. To introduce a new way of doing therapy can be inconvenient to everyone. As an extreme example, a child treatment facility might require psychological testing of the child and an elaborate history and insist that the therapist take extensive process notes of whatever happens. I recall once being asked to comment on a case presented at a private hospital. The client was an 18-year-old who had taken some heroin, apparently to join her boyfriend in this endeavor. I received a 60-page diagnostic report. At the staff meeting I made the comment that an actively oriented therapist would have completed therapy in the time it took to work up this 60-page document. (That comment was not appreciated.) I also pointed out that there was no treatment plan in the document except for the recommendation of the staff that the parents be persuaded to have the young woman hospitalized for a minimum of three years. I talked with the residents after the meeting and learned that the reason for recommending 3 years of hospitalization for the young woman was that that was the length of their training.

What is required for the training context for the approach to supervision recommended here is a setting different from the traditional one. It can be an error to try to supervise someone in a new approach to therapy while in a setting that requires all the old procedures. I have introduced a socially active therapy in a number of agencies over the years, and there are steps that can be taken to make the transition easier.

First of all, the supervisor needs to have the training program approved by the top authorities in the agency. One doesn't want trainees to get caught between a supervisor and an administration that are opposed to each other. The approval should include a few changes: The training program should be freed from the restraints of traditional procedures by creating a unit with its own intake procedures, its own discharge procedures, and its own policy toward making notes on the process of the therapy. The notes, while brief, need to be such that if another therapist picks up the case it would be clear to him or her what had already been done. There should be a one-way mirror and video cameras in the therapy room, and the therapist trainees should be volunteers, not individuals who are required to take the training. The training ideas should not be imposed on staff members who are not in training, but they should be welcome to come and observe the training at any time.

---

[3]See Grove, D., & Haley, J. (1993). *Conversations on therapy.* New York: Norton.

This approach is like a business venture in which an established company creates a new division to develop, test, and market a new product. The process is kept separate from the regular procedures of the company. If the new product is successful, it is absorbed into the larger structure of the company, and if it is not, it is canceled without interfering with the general running of the business. Sometimes a new training program is successful and its principles are adopted by the whole agency; at other times it is expelled, and the agency goes on as it was before.

11

COMPULSORY THERAPY

A young female trainee was given the case of a delinquent boy who had been charged with theft. His parents had been advised that if he went into therapy, the judge would take that as a positive step and not sentence him to jail. The boy came to therapy with his family, which was quite large (it included several siblings and an uncle). The therapist organized the family around the goal of preventing the boy from stealing again. A number of family conflicts came up and were resolved. The family seemed pleased with the therapy, saying they had been able to discuss various concerns for the first time. The therapist was pleased with their cooperation and apparent satisfaction. The court date for the boy was set, and a therapy appointment was made for the following day to discuss what happened and what was to follow. The court, taking into account the family's cooperation by attending therapy, released the young man. The next day the therapist awaited the family to congratulate them on their success. They did not show up or cancel the appointment. When the therapist telephoned, she was rather brusquely informed that the family did not want to come in or have further therapy. The therapist was shocked, realizing that the family had simply used her to avoid a jail sentence for the son. Their cooperation in therapy apparently hadn't been genuine; their attendance at sessions was solely for the purpose of having the therapist advise the court that they had been cooperative in therapy. After this experience, the therapist found herself unable to trust some of her other clients; she worried about simply being used. Her supervisor's task was to prevent this experience from making her cynical and affecting her work in a negative way. It was clear that a new type of therapy had appeared.

Therapy was created to help people who voluntarily seek help, people who have a problem they can't solve themselves. The many schools of therapy are all based on the idea that the client enters therapy voluntarily. Therapists may have different approaches and techniques, but they all assume that their clients are motivated to seek assistance. The voluntary nature of therapy was so taken for granted that it was even argued that people couldn't be helped unless they asked for help. They had to reach bottom to become desperate enough to come in and ask for assistance before they could benefit from therapy. Paying the therapist a fee for help defined therapy as voluntary.

In the last few years a different kind of therapy has appeared. Therapy is now often compulsory. The court system is flooded with a proliferation of abuse cases—neglect and sexual and physical abuse of children, violence between spouses, and substance abuse. Increasing numbers of people are ordered to therapy by judges. The traditional legal penalties for these abuses are sometimes set aside, and therapy is applied to the problem, whether the client wants it or not. Often in such situations, the client doesn't want therapy and the therapist doesn't want to treat a person who doesn't want to be there. Neither one wishes the other's company. This is becoming a familiar context in contemporary therapy.

The discovery of therapy by the legal system has led to various kinds of compulsory treatment. In one type the person is sentenced to go to therapy; it is court ordered. When people are ordered to seek therapy, they have to attend therapy sessions—and pay for them—whether they like it or not. Making people pay for therapy they don't want raises curious ethical issues.

A somewhat less mandatory referral occurs when some representative of the court advises people that it would be a good idea, that the court might smile on them, if they had therapy.

Another version of compulsory therapy is used by people who believe that going into therapy before a trial will increase the possibility of leniency by the judge. These people aren't in therapy to seek help but only to impress the judge. Sometimes they tell their therapist they are in treatment voluntarily and are eager to change, but the therapist learns otherwise when the client simply disappears after the court hearing. Sometimes, however, clients are honest and say they are only in therapy to stay out of jail and have no interest in changing.

Here's an example of an honest client compulsory therapy: A young man sentenced by the court to therapy because of PCP possession and dealing came into therapy with his wife. The therapist met with the couple and asked the man if he would like to change and give up drugs. The man said, "No, I've used them many years, all my life really, and I enjoy it. While I'm having a court ordered urine testing, I'll stay off the stuff, but the day I'm free I'll go back to PCP." The therapist, searching for some way to motivate the man to give up drugs, said, "You know PCP is one of the few drugs that causes brain damage." The man said, "I haven't noticed any brain damage." The therapist turned to the wife for help to increase motivation. He said, "Wouldn't you like to see your husband give up drugs?" The wife replied, "Not really, no." The man said, "She takes more of it than I do. We do it together."

The therapist continued to look for some sort of leverage to encourage reform. At one point the wife said she was thinking about having a baby, and she was a little worried about the effect of drugs on the baby. The therapist looked pleased. He left the room and brought back a pamphlet on the harm drugs do to fetuses. The young man glanced at it and said, "Well, I'm not sure I want a baby."

An exasperated therapist might have rejected this man for therapy, but that would simply have returned the problem to the penal system (which hadn't been successful or it would not be turning to psychotherapy). Or the man might have gone to another therapist and lied rather that tell him the truth.

PARTIALLY COMPULSORY THERAPY

Compulsory therapy is new to supervisors since it is different from the voluntary therapy taught to several generations of therapists in the universities. Yet there has been some experience with partially compulsive therapy. An example is school ordered therapy. When a family comes in with a problem child and is asked, "Why are you here?" they may say, "Because the school told us to come." They don't say, "Because we have a problem that we wish to solve." This type of therapy is compulsory for families in the sense that school can make it difficult for a child if he or she doesn't have therapy. The family comes in only to avoid something worse, which is what defines compulsory therapy.

Every family therapist has also had the experience of seeing family members who come in reluctantly. As far as an adolescent who is dragged into therapy by his or her parents is concerned, the therapy is compulsory therapy. Therapists must find a way to persuade such adolescents that it is really in their best interests to be there. Spouses also come in because one spouse said to the other, "Either we go in or we divorce." Patients in custody in hospitals also experience compulsory therapy. Those of us who have worked in a hospital have had an aide drag a patient to us for a therapy interview, and have said to the patient, "I'm sure tomorrow you will come by yourself." The next day the patient is again unwilling to come, and again the aide drags the patient to therapy. With the power a staff has over patients in a psychiatric hospital, it is sometimes difficult to determine whether the person is voluntarily seeking therapy or not. I am reminded of Erving Goffman's advice to patients on how to get out of a mental hospital: Develop an obvious symptom, talk to the ward psychiatrist about it, and let him "cure" you.

WHOSE AGENT IS THE THERAPIST?

The most important issue in compulsory therapy is the question it raises about whom the therapist represents. A therapist is always the agent of someone. In the early days of therapy the therapist was the agent of an individual client. Such therapists wouldn't even talk to a client's relative on the telephone since they were on the side of the individual in relation to the family (even thought the family was often paying the therapist). At other times the therapist was an agent of the parents against a problem youth. Later, in the period of social change in the 1960s, therapists became the agent of whole families, often siding with the family against the community.

When compulsory therapy is court ordered, the therapist is an agent of the state, a new situation for therapists, at least in the Western world. The fact that therapists help the state make people behave in ways approved by society is an issue those in the therapy field now face. (It is even known that some chapters of Alcoholics Anonymous will report to the court whether a person attends meetings or not. An AA meeting was once the safest place for a person who wished to be anonymous to get help after reaching bottom.) Compulsory therapy is a union of therapy and social control, with the state using therapists to reform troublemakers in these increasingly troubled times. Such clients, for their part, respond to the therapist as an agent of the state. Although many therapists try to persuade the court-ordered client that they represent the client and not the state (even if this is so), the client is naturally uncertain about how much to reveal about his or her illegal acts for fear the therapist will reveal this information to the court. Compulsory therapy can become corrupted and the security of a confidential relationship destroyed not only by the client's fear of revealing personal information to the therapist but also by the therapist's uncertainty about how much he or she must reveal to the court.

The best position for a supervisor to take on compulsory therapy would seem to be to teach that therapists must tell the court whether a court-ordered client shows up for therapy or not and what their recommendation would be. What a client says in the therapy need not be reported to the court.

The extent to which compulsory therapy is used is unknown, but it is on the increase as the court systems turn more and more to therapy as an alternative to incarceration. Not only are therapists now doing compulsory therapy, but there are whole agencies devoted to that practice. One might expect therapists to protest being used in this way, but there has been little protest from them. Most therapists don't like this type of therapy, but unfortunately some of them are pleased by it. A young therapist admitted using confrontational therapy and being pleased that people were ordered to come to him by the court because he could do to them what he wished. Often, drug addicts in groups are put through awful experiences in the name of help. The power of the therapist is increased when the court does the empowering—which is sometimes good and sometimes bad. A new world of treatment is slowly engulfing the field. On a smaller scale, corporations now hire therapists to make workers behave the way the company prefers. These therapists, then, are agents of the corporation, and the employees, who must go to therapy or risk being fired, are clients who are essentially experiencing a form of compulsory therapy.

One problem with compulsory therapy is that there are no organizations of mental health workers discussing the problems involved and no scientific papers being presented that delineate this kind of therapy. People just accept it. Judges who have been sold on the value of therapy often take advantage of it because they don't know what to do with the repeat offenders they must deal with. When an attempt was made to organize a meeting between jurists and therapists on the topic of compulsory therapy, one judge said, "For God's Sake, don't take therapy away from me. I don't know what else to do with these people."

COMPULSORY THERAPY: WHAT IS DIFFERENT?

There are a number of differences between voluntary and compulsory therapy.

Involvement of Other Professionals

In traditional therapy the therapist decides how to conduct therapy treatment. He or she makes the choice of a particular technique and decides which members of the family will be interviewed. The therapist has freedom of choice within the constraints of a particular therapy ideology.

In compulsory therapy a number of professionals are involved in the case, and many of them have more power than the therapist. Involved in the case are police officers, judges, child protective service workers, probation officers, attorneys, and therapists assigned to individual family members. The number of professionals involved makes the case complicated—and sometimes impossible. These professionals have power never previously available in therapy cases. For example, they can take a family member from the home without the therapist's permission. At times a child who is in therapy is taken out of the home without even consultation with the therapist. When family members are removed, the family often doesn't understand why—nor, at times, does the therapist. It is a unique form of family therapy when the therapist cannot even help the family decide who is to live in their home, let alone who is to be present for the family interviews. In one case a therapist had been seeing a family for several months when the sex-abusing father was suddenly taken out of the home. The child protective service workers had finally caught up with the paperwork on the case and were now responding to the situation. The therapist, who felt that all was progressing well, couldn't do a thing about the father being removed.

Family therapy was born when families began to disintegrate in the 1950s. We should acknowledge that therapists and social agencies, could have had much to do with that disintegration inasmuch as their treating individuals and not married couples must have influenced the 50% divorce rate in a negative way. As parents separate, children are often raised in single-parent homes (there are more severe consequences when the dismembered family's children are put in foster homes), older people in increasing numbers are abandoned by their families and put in nursing homes, and adolescents who make trouble are put in psychiatric wards or juvenile halls and treated as individual problems. The family as a unit is becoming dismantled, and we cannot deny that helpful people have contributed to this.

The Need for Rapid Change

The voluntary therapist can choose whether to do therapy quickly or to take time with it as people slowly change. Sometimes an intervention transforms a client immediately, and sometimes the change in a client takes place over time. With abuse cases in compulsory therapy, the therapist doesn't have the option of choosing the length of therapy. If someone is being abused, the therapist must act with a quick intervention. You cannot have a father beating a child a little less each month while the therapist is slowly changing the family. In such cases therapists must act quickly, which is why (along with insurance companies setting time limits) brief therapy workshops are becoming more popular.

The Court's Linear View

Many therapists have attempted to change their thinking from a linear view to a family systems approach to psychopathology. They have given up the idea that human problems have a villain and a victim and believe that what one person does is influenced by what someone else does and that a troubled family follows sequences that keep repeating and that perpetuate distress. For example, they may hypothesize that a misbehaving youth is stabilizing a family through his or her symptom and that this is not a simple matter of bad behavior.

There is a special problem for family therapists who deal with court representatives. The legal system cannot tolerate a system's viewpoint. The court has to be linear and takes a position that there is a villain and a victim. Before a court the individual is responsible for his or her acts and must be punished for committing a crime. It would undermine the whole legal system to allow, for example, the idea that a man steals because his wife provokes him, or that he sexually abused a daughter because a wife neglects or encourages him. An adolescent crime cannot be explained in court as the adolescent's way of helping a depressed parent. If the court allowed a family view of problems, then whole families would need to be put in jail.

When therapists who have a systems view try to collaborate with court representatives who have a linear view, difficulties develop. Court representatives tend to think of family therapists as being too soft on the troubled family members, and family therapists tend to think of court people as being too hard on them. This division of views is typical of the conflict parents have about a problem child.

Belief in Change

Perhaps the most basic difference between therapists and protective service workers results from their social context. The position therapists must take is that change is possible, that whatever the problem, it can be influenced and changed. If abuse occurs in a family, therapists believe a change can take place so that it doesn't occur again. If they didn't believe this, they wouldn't choose a career as a therapist. Therapists also have a responsibility to help the abuser as well as the victim, as part of their larger view of the problem, whereas the court only seeks help for the victim.

In contrast, the safest position for the staff of a child protective agency to take is that change is not likely. If one is protecting a victim, it's best to assume that the abuser will not change and that the abused must be protected forever. If protective service personnel risk the idea that people can change and the abused person is again harmed, they are at fault and must bear the guilt of allowing the abuse. Rather than risk continued abuse, children are separated from the abuser. This is done even though the child might be abused in a foster home or a father might join another family and become abusive with them.

When a therapist who believes change is possible meets a court representative who takes the position that it is not, they have difficulty collaborating with each other. Often, the parties consider it a personal difference when it is really a structural problem in the system. That is, it's because each professional is doing the right thing that the trouble occurs. For example, defense attorneys are employed to protect family members. Attorneys often multiply around an abuse case, with each attorney representing a different member of the family. In one case a brother was arrested for sexually abusing his sister over a period of years. He was given a court-appointed attorney who took the position that he shouldn't say a word about what happened. When the family was ordered to therapy, the son, advised to admit nothing, refused to speak in the family session. His sister, who wanted to protect him, also wouldn't speak. The therapist found it difficult to do therapy with people who refused to communicate. Yet the attorney's position—that the boy should admit nothing if she was to do her job of defending him—was absolutely correct from her point of view. This kind of situation makes it clear that we're not dealing with a simple conflict between professionals. The problem is in trying to blend two very different systems together when there are different concepts of what needs to be done.

The Professional's Emotional Commitment

There are not merely theoretical differences between the professionals involved in abuse cases but powerful emotions as well. Professionals cannot always be rational and objective about an abuse case because their own feelings are caught up in the drama of the situation. This is a special problem for therapists, who are trained to be fair, if not neutral. Every therapist gets upset over a particular kind of abuse; when he or she must work with a case of that particular kind, collaboration *is* difficult.

To cite an example, a 14-year-old girl was sexually abused by her father. He was taken out of the house. The social workers dealing with the case thought the mother was too distant from the daughter, and they encouraged mother and daughter to be closer. A year later the mother began to sexually abuse the child and developed a sexual relationship with her. After a while the mother felt terrible about this and turned herself in. The girl was taken out of her home and put into a shelter, even though she had been a parental child for her three younger siblings. The girl was not even allowed to see her siblings. Nor was the mother permitted to speak to her daughter. When the girl called her mother, her mother would say, "I'm not allowed to speak to you." The girl began to run away from the shelter, once staying out overnight.

A therapist was assigned to the case. He talked with the mother and found her overwhelmed with guilt. The therapist wanted to bring the mother and daughter together to work out what had happened between them, and to help them decide where the daughter should live in the future, as well as other matters, but the protective service people, who were very upset with the mother, refused to allow mother and daughter to be in the same room, even in therapy. A great deal of time was taken up discussing this issue on the telephone. An additional problem was that the woman was very religious. When she confessed to the elders of her church what she had done, they had her shunned by the religious community. Moreover, the members of this religion weren't allowed to make friends outside of the religious group, meaning that this woman couldn't talk to anyone—except her therapist (who was a Catholic priest who was very helpful to her).

The mother's trial date arrived, and she was sentenced to a year in jail. The therapist had to locate a grandmother in a distant city and arrange for her to come and take care of the children. (The father couldn't be brought back into the home since he had been expelled as an abuser.) While the mother was in jail, the daughter was put in a foster home, separated from her family. When the foster mother heard what the mother had done, she was so upset and angry that she spent her time telling the daughter what an awful mother she had.

Meanwhile, the therapist's efforts were directed toward arranging some form of reconciliation between mother and daughter. After long negotiations, protective service workers agreed that mother and daughter could be in the same room with a family therapist provided the daughter also had an individual therapist to support her if she got upset in the family sessions. This was arranged, and at last mother and daughter came together. A session was also arranged so that the daughter could talk to her siblings.

Fortunately, the mother was eventually placed in a prerelease center that was progressive in a number of ways. She did well there: She lost weight, got a job, gained some self-confidence, and continued her therapy. The therapist asked the foster mother to come to a therapy interview since the girl was caught between her and her mother. The foster mother said, "I will never be in the same room with that woman," and she continued telling the girl how awful her mother was.

The mother is now back home, and is continuing to work; the children are doing well. The daughter is still in the foster home. In this case, the vast majority of the therapist's time was used to deal with other professionals, which seems typical in compulsory therapy cases when the abuse is particularly upsetting to the therapist.

THE FUTURE OF COMPULSORY THERAPY

The field of therapy is always changing and taking on new forms and procedures. It appears that it will even absorb compulsory therapy. It would be an easier transition if some simple steps could be taken: One step should be to have training programs that teach therapists ways to motivate clients who don't choose to be in therapy. Such training should help therapists avoid being an agent of the state and should teach them how to be an agent of the client while acknowledging the needs of the community.

At present, each therapist is struggling with these problems in isolation and attempting to devise procedures to deal with them. Some therapists seem to have little or no difficulty with compulsory therapy cases while others have awful problems. Some have developed special techniques. For example, it is helpful in the first 15 minutes of a first family interview with a compulsory case to have a court representative explain the legal situation, which in many cases was previously unintelligible to the family. After thanking and dismissing the court representative the therapist can turn to the family and say something like, "What a difficult problem we face." At that point the state is gone out of the room and the therapist is on the side of the family. Supervisors should develop a variety of such simple procedures for trainees to help them deal with compulsory therapy cases.

What's also needed is some kind of forum in each community where court representatives and therapists can meet together and discuss the issues related to the cases they share. Differences could be worked out in an atmosphere of unhurried deliberation which is difficult to achieve in a brief telephone call, which is how collaboration seems to occur now. It might also be helpful if a different term could be substituted for *compulsory therapy*—for example, *court counseling*, or *court practice*—to distinguish it from the kind of enterprise in which a therapist promotes the growth of people who have done nothing wrong.

Finally, it would be helpful if judges who assign cases to therapists would also require a scientific follow-up to determine if, in fact, therapy is more successful than jail in terms of the frequency of recidivism. It might be that therapy is a great success with compulsory cases—or it might not be. We should know because important civil liberties are at stake.

Epilogue
HOW TO BE A THERAPY SUPERVISOR WITHOUT KNOWING HOW TO CHANGE ANYONE

Therapy trainees, like flocks of doves, flutter in increasing numbers from universities and private training institutes. All of these therapists must be trained by supervisors. Where can competent supervisors be found who know how to change people? Without enough trained supervisors, particularly in a brief and family-oriented therapy, there is a crises. Young therapists in the field must change clients who won't eat, are on drugs, won't stop crying, are acting crazy, are abusing children, are attempting suicide, are afraid, or can't stop behaving in foolish ways. The desperate trainee turns to a supervisor and says, "What should I do to cure these people?" Supervisors who were never taught what to do with such problems experience difficulty. Vast numbers of trainees are being taught by supervisors who know how to reflect on life's problems but do not know what to do to solve those problems. In the last few years therapy has changed to an active, directive style partly because the

A variation of this article was previously published in the *Journal of Systemic Therapies* (1993, Fall), 4–52.

insurance industry and the courts require that therapy be brief and that a successful outcome be evident. Those who manage care expect supervisors to teach a short-term therapy, telling trainees what to do to solve therapy problems and how to do it quickly. Generations of therapy supervisors were taught that therapy and supervision are leisurely inquiries featuring reflection rather than action. They were not trained to solve a client's problem but to discuss other matters, like why people are the way they are and how they got that way. As Al Titicaca, Ph.D. (not his real name), said, "I can establish a good relationship with a trainee, and we can have a productive talk about personal problems, how to make process notes, and the dynamics and childhood origins of a case. Then the trainee asks me what to do with a client who won't ever take a bath. I talk about the deeper meanings of bathing, but I don't really have any idea what to do." A female supervisor, Virginia (her real name), said, "I was supervising a therapist with a client who compulsively sang 'The Star-Spangled Banner' every time she had an orgasm. I simply didn't know what to do to help her over that embarrassing problem despite my years of training as a supervisor. I can join therapists in a feminist perspective, and I can discuss systems theory at length, but when they want to know what to do to change someone, I'm just lost and have to call upon my experience at faking it."

Most supervisors are like Al and Virginia, in need of help to conceal the fact that they don't know how to change people. Guidelines are offered here for making use of basic supervision techniques that have helped teachers conceal ignorance for generations. These include arranging the proper context, offering the correct presentation of self, and recognizing that the different clinical theories were designed not so much to guide therapists as to help supervisors who don't know what to do.

THE IMPORTANCE OF PROPER CONTEXT

The supervisor can take comfort in the fact that the social context frames all statements. Just being in a supervisory job means that one is assumed to be knowledgeable. If a supervisor can find employment in a well-known institution, even banal comments are thought profound. A dumb statement in a wise context, such as Harvard University, will be admired, as many dumb teachers there have found. It helps if the supervisor explains that he or she is descended from a distinguished line of supervisors. Attending weekend workshops featuring famous, even legendary, supervisors means one can identify them as former teachers and refer to them by their first names. It is also important to be properly licensed and to display these awards prominently in one's office. Certification as an approved supervisor is not difficult to obtain: It only requires paying a fee, attending classes, writing papers, and talking about dynamics. Evidence that the supervisor has successfully taught trainees any therapy techniques, such as skill in the use of various interventions, is not required.

THE PRESENTATION OF SELF

How should supervisors present themselves when facing a class of beginning trainees? It is best to present one's self as having a flavor of both wisdom and wit. If only half of either quality is present, the condition can be concealed by a thoughtful manner. A contemplative personal style—as if one is always considering all aspects of every situation—should be cultivated. Supervisors must appear to have what the title implies, namely, "super vision." Two vision mannerisms are helpful: (1) a faraway look that implies one is considering all aspects of the larger situation, and (2) a keen incisive look that shows the student that one is alert and quickly grasping the essentials. When a nervous student is worried about the fate of the client in his or her hands, the supervisor can win respect and even adulation just by being there, remaining calm, and looking wise. The faraway look and thoughtful silence can, at times, cause the trainee to become impatient enough to come up with an idea of something to do. The supervisor can accept the trainee's idea, perhaps implying that he or she had that very thing in mind and merely wanted the trainee to think of it spontaneously. If a student already has a plan and is seeking approval for it, a sharp, knowing look by the supervisor is correct even if he or she doesn't understand the plan.

The proper manner alone cannot prevent students from being critical. One must develop a personal relationship with trainees so that they will have such loyalty that they minimize, or even overlook, one's deficiencies. Generally, it helps if the supervisor can remember a student's name. Occasional personal comments are also important, for example, "I understand your wife had triplets this morning. Well done." It is personal involvement that encourages students to be uncritical, even protective, of the incompetent supervisor.

With the correct manner in an impressive context, a supervisor can win the respect of trainees even without knowing how to induce therapeutic change. However, what if the supervisor is specifically asked what to do to change a client with a serious problem? There are accepted ways to deal with this crisis. The most popular way is to behave like a cognitive therapist and obscure issues by rationally discussing theory. It's no longer a secret that the basic ideologies of therapy were designed to protect supervisors who don't know what to do to bring about change.

THE IDEAL THEORY

Let us examine the criteria of a clinical theory that would be ideal for supervisors who don't know how to bring about change. Such a theory would need to address the following issues:

First, is it possible to arrange that a supervisor cannot fail? That sounds difficult, but wise heads have applied themselves for the last century and provided solutions. What if, after completing training, a student hasn't changed a single client and lacks all skill except the ability to say, "Tell me more about that"? Can a supervisor avoid being blamed as a failure?

Second, how can a supervisor avoid having to innovate different therapy techniques for each case? If one could devise a single method simple enough for any teacher to understand and explain to trainees, no one would expect teachers to devise unique interventions.

Third, if a supervisor is ignorant of how to bring about change, what can he or she talk about that would distract trainees from therapy issues? It should be something interesting and intriguing to fascinate young intellectual types so that they won't notice that they are not being taught how to change real problems.

Fourth, can a supervisor not have anything expected of him or her for years and so avoid criticism until the issues, and the case, no longer matter?

Fifth, can one arrange that a supervisor is never proven wrong? In the ideal teaching situation this is the most important task. A trainee might say bitterly, "After years of therapy under your supervision I haven't accomplished anything in the way of change in this client, and you have never given me any help." The teacher needs to respond so that the trainee slinks away, chastened and ashamed for having been critical and for making foolish demands on the supervisor.

In summary, the ideal situation for a supervisor would be one with no responsibility for change, no risk of being wrong, and no risk of criticism. Is it too much to expect this ideal to be found anywhere in the real world? We must turn to the classic schools of therapy to discover how this ideal has been achieved. We will find that the primary purpose of the powerful procedures and ideologies of the therapy field is to help supervisors who don't know how to bring about change.

PAST AND PRESENT THEORIES

Examining classical theories isn't of merely historical interest but can actually be a discussion of contemporary psychotherapy. Generations of therapists were trained in those ideas, and supervisors today practice as their teachers did. Therapy techniques may change out in the field, but supervision procedures to protect incompetent teachers never change.

It is well known that the therapies with the least practical value and poorest outcome are based on psychodynamic theory. Yet those ideas are still a popular set in the field today. Why is that? Obviously, it's not coincidence that (1) the theory is perpetuated by supervisors and that (2) it is the theory that is more protective of incompetent teachers than any theory yet devised. Contemporary contributions offer only modifications.

Before the turn of the last century, in that great period of hypnotic therapy, Freud went about visiting the hypnotherapists of his day. What he observed was live supervision of therapy. A supervisor would demonstrate hypnotic therapy with a patient, focusing on the symptom the person wished to recover from. The trainee would watch the hypnotic expert solve the problem. After observing the teacher, the trainee would work with a patient and solve a problem while the teacher watched. This live supervision was based on the assumption that training in how to do therapy involves the teaching of a skill.

After watching these hypnotherapists at work and trying it himself, Freud decided to give up hypnosis and take a very different approach. The only explanation for this change is that he must have said to himself, "The fellows I work with could never teach therapy this way. They couldn't invent a strategy for each case. They could never demonstrate such skill in curing new symptoms and so couldn't teach that to trainees. Therefore, I must develop another form of therapy, one that allows teachers to have prestige and be admired even when they don't know how to bring about change. Can I build an organization based on this principle?"

After long hours of meditation, perhaps sitting nose to nose with his friend and consultant Wilhelm Fliess, Freud came up with the classic approach that is still in daily use 100 years later. It's a tribute to Freud that he achieved every requirement in our fantasy about how to save incompetent teachers. So great is his influence that his supervisory ideas are used today even by teachers of different therapies with new and more fashionable names.

HOMAGE TO FREUD

Freud went to the heart of the matter at once by proposing a two-pronged approach to save the teacher. He devised a form of therapy in which the therapist, and therefore the supervisor, didn't take responsibility for changing anyone. He added the idea that any failure of the trainee is the fault of the trainee's emotional problems, not the failure of his or her teacher. With these two basic assumptions, any incompetent supervisor could divert the slings and arrows of outraged trainees who might notice that they are failing to change anyone.

If a patient says, "Isn't it your job to change me?" the traditional therapist is taught to reply, "No, my job is to help you understand yourself. Whether or not you change is up to you." This has been acknowledged as a way to arrange that therapists need not know what to do. Overlooked is the fact that this instruction contains a covert agenda for the supervisor. If trainees say the same thing to their supervisor—for example, "Isn't it your job to tell me how to get this client over his misery?"—the supervisor can respond, "It's not my job to help you change people but to help you understand why you have problems in dealing with this patient." The supervisor can even give a smile of derision and inquire about the trainee's unresolved emotional problems. "Have you examined your omnipotent fantasies of saving patients?" the supervisor can ask, and the embarrassed trainees will drag themselves away to deal with their emotional problems, not noticing that their teacher didn't know how to solve the client's problem. The blame of the trainee's own problems also persuades the trainee to be a person who distrusts his or her judgments rather than one who criticizes the teacher.

As part of Freud's schema, he did away with live supervision and insisted that therapy be confidential. It should be done in private offices with double doors so that no one can watch or hear anyone say or do anything, even when leaning against the door. In this way teachers need not demonstrate their skill to trainees or observe techniques of interviewing by trainees. Trainees who lack skill cannot be held responsible if no one ever sees them do an interview.

Freud's second step was to insist on a single method. The supervisor teaches that the patient should do all the talking while the therapist only asks an occasional question (this is called "making an interpretation"). The insightful interpretation is the invariant prescription that distracts the client into wondering why he or she has the problem rather than what to do about it.

Great emphasis was put on being nondirective. The argument was offered that telling people to do anything—except lie down and talk to the ceiling—was demeaning to them and would interfere with the goals of neutrality. It was argued that only a one-way monologue caused change. In this way supervisors could avoid having to learn how to give directives and how to determine which ones to use for particular problems.

A third step to save teachers from knowing how to cure symptoms was to say that symptoms are unimportant and that what should be discussed is what's behind, or around the corner from, them. Since this innovation created a therapy without goals, no supervisor can be faulted if the trainee doesn't achieve a goal.

Supervisors were especially helped because therapy was designed to be long term. Years passed and generations passed away before a therapy was over. How could anyone know whether the case, and therefore the supervisor, had failed?

With two more prongs Freud, who was fond of a prong, solved the question of (1) what interesting topic could be talked about and (2) how a supervisor could never be proven wrong. He proposed that therapy should never deal with the real, only the fantasy, world. There is a current controversy over why Freud gave up the issue of sexual abuse of his young female patient in the real world and turned it into a wish, or fantasy, that lurked in the dark recesses of their minds. What should a therapist do about an incestuous father? According to Freud, one should say nothing happened. Apparently, he wished to save his teachers from having to deal with reality, where they could be proven wrong and would have to know what to do about real people, like horny relatives. When talking about a fantasy instead of facts, who can say the supervisor is right or wrong?

What about the major challenge, namely how to distract the trainee from the issue of how to change people by having the supervisor talk about something else really interesting? Look what Freud, in his genius, provided: He not only presented an intriguing explanation of human motivation and new ways of seeing human kind but focused his training on all the most exciting issues in life. He recommended that the teacher talk about sex, power, conflict, the envy of different types of genitalia, and the stark human dramas of fantasies of murder and incest. Does the boy have a secret passion for his mother? Does the daughter get electrified with desire for her father? All else seems idle talk in the face of such dramatic issues. Choosing to talk about what normal people would censor as unmentionable, Freud ensured that supervisory sessions were endlessly titillating. Each consultation with a supervisor was an adventure in awfulness. How to change people could be overlooked as a side issue.

Freud managed to achieve every single one of the ideal ways to protect incompetent teachers. In addition, he persuaded everyone that conversation and not action is what therapists should do. Therapy supervisors have been benefactors of his ideas for a century. Even new therapies with different ideologies continue to base the training of therapists on Freud's principles for saving supervisors.

UP WITH DIAGNOSIS

Of course we need not give all credit to Freud. Other schools of therapy have added ways to save supervisors. We need not dwell on how supervisors are protected with the approach of Carl Rogers. They only teach the therapist to reflect back what the client says. Most supervisors can manage that.

The value of diagnosis for the supervisor who doesn't know what to do is well known. Rather than talk about therapy, it was discovered that hours of supervision time can be used up discussing the proper diagnosis. Dwelling on the DSM-IV, the supervisor who discovers that a client fits into a category, or even three or four of them, will arouse an excited feeling of accomplishment in the trainee. "Clearly a borderline personality and not a schizoid state," says the supervisor. "Gosh!" says the trainee in admiration. It takes time doing therapy in the real world before the therapist notices that the diagnostic system is irrelevant and even a handicap to changing people.

When supervisors train psychiatric residents today, diagnosing and choosing a drug, or even three or four, are the only activities. A record for talking about medication was established by a group in the University of Iowa Department of Psychiatry. They are reported to have talked for 2 hours and 38 minutes about which medication should be used to defeat the unfortunate side effects of Haldol, which had been given to a woman when she complained of anxiety while bungee-jumping off the Tallahatchie Bridge.

NEW TIMES

As times change, something new for supervisors is becoming necessary. Let us outline the challenge: Many protective procedures of supervisors are being abandoned just when more supervisors are being trained. Confidentiality, the key protection for supervisors, is being threatened with the development of the one-way mirror and the audio and video recording of interviews. The supervisor's lack of knowledge is put on public display instead of being shown only to one supervisee in confidence. Live supervision requires that a teacher know how to guide a trainee during an actual therapy interview, not later when the discussion can only be about what might have been. Because of the popularity of live supervision, it is the lucky supervisor who can avoid the one-way mirror.

Therapists are also under great pressure to know what to do about presenting problems. A reliance on the past and on fantasies is being given up as the real world of clients is discovered to be a pain. At the same time, social changes are occurring and the poor and new ethnic groups are descending upon therapists. Traditionally, therapists were impatient with the poor and refused to treat them since they wouldn't come on time or pay their bills regularly. Supervisors needed only to have keen insight into the middle classes; now they must deal with poor people as well as with members of 180 ethnic groups, many of whom do not even speak English. Therapy is also being applied to more difficult problems, such as violence, suicide, rape, drug abuse, incest, criminal activities, and other troubling behaviors. To deal with these unfortunate people, therapists have to know what they're doing. Supervisors who don't know how to teach what to do are under attack. The latest complication for supervisors is the discovery that therapists and clients come in two genders. Feminist therapists protest past and present biases and blame supervisors. How can supervisors conceal incompetence and sexism when all is visible and the focus is on actual people in the real world? Can that challenge be met? Let us discuss how theory can be helpful, as always.

MODERN THEORY

One way to salvage the supervisor with theory is to provide a theory so complex that no one can understand it, not even a supervisor. This is what happened with the theory of family therapy. Alternatively, one can provide a theory so simple that any supervisor, no matter how dumb, can understand it. This is what happened with the theory of behavior therapy. Pavlov discovered that if a creature is rewarded for doing something, it will do more of that something. If it's punished for doing something, it will do less of that something. To this remarkable finding was added the idea that if people are holding their noses when they are punished, they will get uneasy whenever they touch their noses. (This has been one explanation of the concern with noses of Freud's friend Fliess.) Skinner leaped upon this theory and expanded the ideas slightly. On that rock was built the church of behavior therapy, a system most teachers could grasp.

Family therapists took quite the opposite approach, seeking more complexity. They created theories so complicated that no teacher could be expected to understand them. Fortunately, there was a giant brain in the field whose ability to be ambiguous was legendary: Gregory Bateson, who became the theoretician of family therapy. Although not particularly interested in therapy, he, along with Don Jackson, introduced the idea of homeostasis into the field and applied that view to whole families he began to interview on his research project. This cybernetic view allows teachers to confound trainees with a complex set of ideas about governed systems, feedback processes, step functions, and negative entropy, all wrapped up in the second law of thermodynamics. Trainees try to conceal the fact that they don't understand the theory and so don't notice that their teachers don't understand it either. It's not necessary for the teachers to teach how to change anyone because the theory is about how systems correct themselves and do not change. European intellectuals like this theory because they believe that changing is actually not changing because it is all constructivist. Americans tend to be more pragmatic and practical, and so they are just confused. A new discovery was recently made that has resulted in a change in the cybernetics of family therapy: third-order change. First-order cybernetics was the discovery that family members respond to each other. Second-order cybernetics was Harry Stack Sullivan's discovery that there is a therapist involved in the observation and that he or she influences the data. Third-order cybernetics is the discovery that supervisors need cybernetic theory to conceal the fact that they don't know how to change anyone.

When Bateson died, systems theory was in danger of becoming more understandable. However, sophisticated theoreticians, faced with the threat of having to know how to do therapy, leaped in to offer complex theories of aesthetic epistemologies with dissociated states with narratives based on constructivist principles. Teachers could continue to avoid teaching how to bring about change and be wise and impenetrable. The post of Chief of Ambiguity is still open and eagerly sought by many contenders. There are two main schools in the competition: One is the "tom-tom" school, whose theme song is a tale of Hoffman and which prides itself on following a different, soundless drum; the hope of leaders of this school is to find a foreign philosopher somewhere who will make them wise. Another school is called the "gray is not white no matter what anybody says" school. It is difficult to find since it is becoming more and more obscure. When a trainee asks what to do to change someone in therapy, a supervisor of this school may respond with the following quote.

> The constitutionalist perspective that I am arguing for refutes foundationalist assumptions of objectivity, essentialism and representationalism. It proposes that an objective knowledge of the world is not possible, that knowledges are actually generated in particular discursive fields. It proposes that all essentialist notions, including those about human nature, are ruses that disguise what is really taking place, that essentialist notions are paradoxical in that they provide descriptions that are specifying of life; that these notions obscure the operations of power. And the constitutionalist perspective proposes that the descriptions that we have of life are not representations or reflections of life as lived, but are directly constitutive of life; that these descriptions do not correspond with the world, but have real effect in the shaping of life. [The reader is challenged to find the source of this quote. It is on page 125 of a book that is better avoided.]

We can only admire this example since it shows that therapy can always produce major theoreticians to obscure the issues and save supervisors.

Still, what is to be done with trainees who persist in saying, "Bosh to theory. What do I do to stop a man from beating his wife and molesting his five children?" Family therapy forces attention on the real world, and trainees expect supervisors to tell them something practical to do. The family emphasis risks clarity, but fortunately it also touches on sensitive issues for trainees who are still disengaging from their own families and wondering if they are dysfunctional. Discussing parents and children and in-laws is always highly charged with personal biases and memories of mistreatment. By dwelling on the personal experience of the trainees, supervisors can distract them from concerns about how one causes change.

The most popular approach with families continues to be the emphasis on the individual. Each year the individual is said to be rediscovered, especially by supervisors who never lost him. An alternate objection that comes up each year is that it's improper to plan what the therapist is to do because advance planning is power oriented. If the therapist just goes to the interview without preconceptions and hopes to find out what might be relevant to something, this approach is more spontaneous and not coercive. A new objection is to say that the one-way mirror is undemocratic and that all the therapists should be pals with the family and join them in the interview room. This is a way for the supervisor to avoid needing to be an expert who knows what to do. Of course, it is hoped that the disagreements among the professionals will not escalate and will somehow transform the clients.

AVOIDING THE NEED TO TEACH SKILLS

When we look objectively at family therapy training, we notice that there has not been a new contribution to save teachers. Even though doing a new form of therapy, most family therapy training programs simply make use of past ideas of training. The primary way trainees are taught in family therapy is to focus on themselves in personal therapy or with the use of family histories in the form of genograms. However, the language is more contemporary. For example, one enthusiast put it this way: "Training in systems awareness calls the attention of trainees to the resonances from level to level of continuous systems. The resonances with one's most intimate person produces the sharpest learning curve." (This quote can be found hidden in an advertisement for family therapy training, published in an appropriate place.)

Some supervisors know how to interview a family and explore problems but don't know how to change them. When such interviews are objected to as being irrelevant to changing people, one solution for a supervisor is to prove that such interviews are important by bringing in guest interviewers for public demonstrations to the trainees. These national teachers are sometimes called "master therapists" by the people organizing the workshops. Apparently, the organizers call anyone who ever spoke in public a master therapist. To distinguish teachers from therapists, a way must be found to differentiate a master therapist from a "legendary supervisor" (defined as someone who has spoken in public more than once). On the national scene these legendary supervisors demonstrate the interviewing of families in front of crowds. Thousands of young people have learned to interview families before a large crowd, if they can only find one.

STEALING IDEAS

Is it possible for contemporary supervisors to provide the trainee with solutions to problems without themselves having to think of any? Does that seem too much to ask? Fortunately, supervisors have found a way.

If one cannot think of a solution to the client's problem, an obvious thing to do is to ask the client for a solution and use that. This is called "solution stealing therapy." It is easier to teach this procedure to therapists than to teach them to innovate solutions of their own. There are two opposite approaches: One is to ask clients what they have tried to do to solve their problem and then to tell them to go ahead and do more of that. The other is to ask clients what solutions they have tried and then tell them that what they tried didn't work but that a slight modification of their solution will solve their problem. This is called the "client must be wrong or he or she wouldn't have a problem but still I can borrow that solution" approach. In this way the supervisor need not think of any new solution but only swipes the one the client offers.

Is there any other possibility to save supervisors who cannot come up with a solution or a therapeutic plan? If supervisors could just tell people to stay the way they are, they wouldn't need to think of anything new for them to do. This innovation has been introduced by contemporary supervisors. It is called "paradox" and is commonly used in therapy, but usually its value to the supervisor is not discussed.

A paradoxical intervention is one where therapists direct clients to continue as they have been in situations where they are asking for a change. They are told to continue with their symptom, as couples are told to maintain the marital quarrel, and families are encouraged to do whatever they've been doing that results in distress. It seems apparent at once that this technique must have been developed for teachers who could not think of what to teach a trainee to do. A supervisor need only teach trainees to tell the client families to stay as they are. It is evident that supervisors on the lower scales of intelligence can grasp that intervention.

CONCLUSION

As we look back over the past 20 years, it would seem evident that therapy training in its many forms has largely borrowed from the past and has not introduced new ways to save the therapy teacher who doesn't know what to do. After all, there have always been obscure theories, paradox, personal therapy, and demonstration interviews.

Someone, perhaps a naive trainee, might ask, "Why save the incompetent supervisor?" Why protect the teacher who doesn't know how to change people? Shouldn't we encourage trainees to rebel against the incompetent? When considering such a reckless plan, let us examine one aspect of training that has been forced upon us with the advent of family therapy and systems theory. It has become apparent that what happens in the training program happens in the therapy. That is, what happens behind the one-way mirror duplicates what happens in front of the mirror (even if there is no mirror). If incompetent trainees are excused by saying that they have emotional problems, the same idea will be fostered in client families, whose members will excuse each other in the same way. If insight is imposed upon trainees in the observation room, it is also imposed by trainees upon the families in the therapy room. If trainees accuse each other with interpretations about their awful psychopathology, as found in the DSM-IV, family members, in street language, can accuse each other of curious categories of abnormal psychology. When supervisor and trainees are pals and humanistic together with democratic teams mirroring each other, the family in therapy will lose its structure and its hierarchy will become disorganized. Hierarchies mirror hierarchies in the therapy field, as the neoconstructivists insist.

How is this relevant to saving supervisors? If training programs don't protect incompetent supervisors but encourage trainees to disrespect them and even laugh at them because they don't know how to change people, what happens to the families in therapy? On the family side of the mirror all authority will be ridiculed, causing confusion everywhere as helpless parents become more so. If respect is to be maintained for, and among, clients every training project must respect and protect the many inadequate teachers.

At the moment, there are increasing numbers of dissatisfied therapy trainees who protest that they aren't learning how to do therapy and who even seek to avoid their supervisors. What can be done? An ideal solution would be to make it illegal for trainees not to listen to supervisors. As a matter of fact, that is now being arranged. The powerful lobbyists who represent professional organizations have persuaded legislators that a therapist must be licensed by them to earn an income. Anyone who does therapy without a license is breaking the law. To gain the license, the therapist must listen to a supervisor and pay for the privilege. So now the law requires therapists to listen to supervisors if they are ever going to make a living. The supervisor, too, must be certified, but fortunately that does not require much. Showing success in teaching therapists how to induce change is not required; all that is needed is many hours of therapist and supervisor sitting and talking together. Any supervisor with a comfortable chair and healthy vocal chords can manage that.

Fortunately, the number of supervisors who know how to change people is increasing, and we can hope that this fortunate trend will continue. Those who don't know what to do will continue to surmount that obstacle in ways that previous generations have used. Large numbers of supervisors of therapy are respected and revered and even have establish new schools of therapy, although they are not teaching anyone how to change anyone no how, in no way, with no problem, of no kind.

INDEX

229